How To Color Your Hair At Home

Just Like A Professional

© 1991 by Doris Möller
All rights reserved.
No part of this book may be reproduced in any form without permission.

Published by Rosetree Publishing Inc.

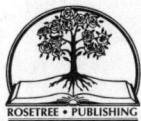

204 Glebeholme Blvd.
Toronto, Ontario M4J 1S9
Tel: (416) 975-1737
Fax: (416) 539-8533

Note: The author and publisher assume no liability whatsoever for any loss or damage resulting from the application of the products or the methods described herein.

Contents

Introduction ... 5
- What This Book Can Do For You ... 6
- How To Use This Book ... 6
- Why Product Instructions Are Not Enough ... 7

Getting Started
- A Plan For Coloring Your Hair ... 8
- Setting Up To Color Your Hair At Home ... 9
- Hair Coloring Accessories ... 11
- Buying Hair Color In The Drugstore ... 12
- Which Brand Of Hair Color Should You Buy? ... 13

Selecting The Right Color
- Why It Is Important To Know The Color Level of Your Hair Before Coloring Your Hair ... 14
- How You Can Determine Your Hair Color Level ... 15
- Chart Of Hair Color Levels and Tones ... 16
- Know Your Color-Type: Choosing The Hair Color That Suits You ... 16
- The Four Color-Types And How Their Hair Can Be Colored ... 23

Selecting And Applying Hair Color
- Types Of Hair Colors: To What Extent They Can Change Your Natural Hair Color ... 24
- Selecting Between Temporary Rinses, Semi-Permanent Rinses, Permanent Hair Color And Bleach ... 25
- Temporary Rinse ... 25
- When To Use A Temporary Rinse ... 25
- How To Apply A Temporary Rinse ... 27
- Other Temporary Colors ... 28
- Semi-Permanent Hair Color - Category I ... 30
- When To Use A Semi-Permanent Rinse ... 30
- How To Choose Your Color ... 30
- What A Semi-Permanent Rinse Cannot Be Used For ... 32
- How To Apply A Semi-Permanent Hair Color ... 33

Contents

- Choosing The Right Semi-Permanent Hair Color Tone For Your Color-Type — **34**
- Semi-Permanent Hair Color - Category II (Long-Lasting) — **35**
- Choosing The Right Long-Lasting Semi-Permanent Rinse Tone — **35**
- How To Apply A Long-Lasting Semi-Permanent Hair Color — **37**
- Henna — **39**
- Choosing The Right Henna Tone For Your Color-Type — **40**
- Permanent Hair Color (Tint) — **41**
- When To Use A Permanent Hair Color — **41**
- How To Apply A Tint — **43**
- Important Points To Remember When Tinting Your Hair — **49**
- Metallic Hair Dye — **51**
- Bleach (Pre-Lightening) — **52**
- How To Apply A Bleach — **53**
- Testing For Allergic Reactions — **57**
- How To Test Your New Hair Color — **58**

Techniques The Professionals Use
- Tinting White/Grey Hair Red — **60**
- How To Highlight Your Hair — **61**
- The Two-Step Method For Coloring Your Hair Light Blonde — **66**
- Low Lighting — **68**
- Coloring Your Light Blonde Bleached Or Tinted Hair Back To Its Natural Color — **70**
- Customizing Your Hair Color — **72**
- Examples Of Mixing Two Different Hair Colors — **73**
- Know A Little Bit Of Color Theory — **74**

Contents

Correcting Undesirable Hair Colors
- How To Correct Undesirable Hair Colors   **76**
- Correcting Hair Color That Is Too Dark After Using A Permanent Hair Color   **76**
- Correcting Dark Ends On Tinted Hair   **82**
- Correcting A Brassy/Reddish Hair Color   **84**
- Correcting A Hair Color That Is Too Gold/Brassy   **85**
- Correcting A Hair Color That Is Too Yellow   **86**
- Correcting Tinted Hair That Has Become "Green"   **87**
- Correcting The Hair Color Of Light Blonde Hair   **88**
- How To Remove Henna From Your Hair   **89**
- How To Remove Metallic Dyes From Your Hair   **90**

Answers To 10 Common Questions
- Can Coloring Your Hair Damage Your Hair?   **92**
- The Chemistry Of Your Hair   **93**
- What Does pH Mean?   **94**
- Why Do Permanent Hair Colors And Bleaches Need To Be Alkaline?   **96**
- Can A Tint Make Your Hair Fall Out?   **97**
- Processing Time For Hair Color: How Important Is It?   **98**
- How You Can Tell How Much White/Grey Hair You Have   **99**
- Perming Colored Hair   **99**
- How Often Should You Tint Your Hair?   **100**
- How To Care For Colored Hair   **100**

Glossary   **101**

Introduction

This book is written for men and women who are already coloring their own hair or who would like to color their own hair but lack the confidence. Although most commercial hair color is marketed for women, these hair coloring products are equally suitable for men. There is absolutely no difference between mens' and womens' hair. Any kind of hair - fine, coarse, straight or curly - can be colored. Hair coloring products sold in drugstores are the essentially same ones sold to hair salons and there is no difference between hair colors for men and women. The only thing that is different is the packaging and the marketing. Over the years, hair colors have become very easy to use. However, whenever you attempt to do anything that is totally different and unfamiliar, from painting and wallpapering your house to coloring your hair, you owe it to yourself to get to know the basics first.

Introduction

What This Book Can Do For You

This book is aimed at taking the guesswork out of hair coloring by showing you what to do, how to do it, when to do it and why it needs to be done in a certain way. It will give you the confidence to color your own hair by providing you with the necessary knowledge to do it correctly. The chances of getting unwanted results will be eliminated when you follow the instructions and guidelines contained in this book. You will also save time and money. Getting your hair color done by a "professional" hair colorist will cost anywhere between $25 to $100, whereas coloring your own hair will cost you between $5 and $15. What's more, you will feel a sense of freedom and accomplishment.

How To Use This Book

Let's assume that you want to do something different with your hair color. Perhaps you find your hair color boring. Or perhaps you find that the grey hair that is showing through more and more is making you look older. You can sense that a change in hair color would make you look much better. "But how", you ask yourself. "What do I have to do first? Where do I start? "It's all so new and you're afraid to make a mistake. You will find that three questions will come to your mind.

1) What color (shade) is the right one for me
2) What kind of hair color should I buy
3) How do I put the color on properly.

Even though every page in this book is filled with useful information for the person who wants to color his/her hair, I suggest that first you read the sections that answer these major questions - questions that inevitably need answering if you are thinking of changing the color of your hair.

The easiest and fastest way to use the information presented in this book is to read the following sections first, where the three basic questions for coloring your hair will be answered: "Selecting The Right Color", pages 14 to 23, "Selecting And Applying Hair Color", pages 24 to 59, "A Plan For Coloring Your Hair", pages 8, "Techniques The Professionals Use", pages 60 to 75, "Answers To 10 Common Questions", pages 90 to 100, "Correcting Undesirable Hair Colors", pages 76 to 91.

Introduction

Why Product Instructions Are Not Enough

The directions that accompany a hair coloring product are kept as basic as possible to ensure that the consumer understands how to use the product. Although hair coloring is not a complicated subject, it is still to your advantage to know basic hair coloring principles and techniques. Questions concerning hair coloring techniques are not answered in the product instructions, often making coloring your hair a matter of trial and error. However it is not the manufacturers' responsibility to teach you the subject of hair coloring. Their job is to tell you how to use their particular product. The rest depends on your own knowledge and judgement.

So here is what you need to know to successfully color your hair at home…

Getting Started

A Plan For Coloring Your Hair

It is often recommended that the best way to start coloring your hair is to use a temporary rinse or a semi-permanent rinse (non-permanent hair color) in order to "try out" a hair color. However, different hair colors have specialized uses. Some cover white hair well whereas others don't. You shouldn't have to experiment, but instead have a plan for how you are going to color your hair.

First read this book carefully. Then ask yourself the following question: "Why do I want to color my hair?" The answer might be that you want to cover your grey hair and/or make your own hair color more interesting. Next, you will need to determine:

1. The color of your hair.
2. Your color type.
3. The type of hair color you want to use.
4. The shade and tone you want to use.
5. How to apply the hair color correctly.

Go over the list of "Setting up to Color your Hair at Home" on page 9 and make a list of items you will need to buy in the drugstore. Reading this book will give you answers to the above questions with which you can make a plan to color your hair.

For instance, let's say that 50% of your hair is grey and you want to color it. However, you want to color it the same color as your own dark hair. Before going out to buy your hair color you will need to have the following type of information. For example:

1. My hair color is light brown.
2. I am a strong-cool color-type (winter).
3. The type of hair color I need to use is a permanent color.
4. The shade I want to use is a light ash brown.
5. Since this is the first time I am coloring my hair, I can use an applicator bottle to apply the color on my hair.

You are now in control. You will no longer have to leave your color choice to fate. You are now ready to head for the permanent hair color

Getting Started

section in the drugstore where you will verify your color on the color selection chart, buy light ash brown and any other items (such as an applicator bottle etc.) you need.

NOTE: Although the hair coloring kit comes with its own applicator bottle, using a professional type applicator bottle is preferable. This applicator bottle has a longer nozzle, is more flexible and being transparent allows you to see how much color you have left.

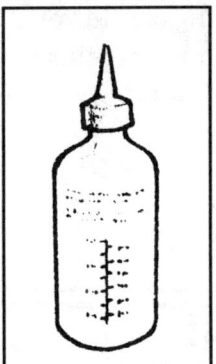

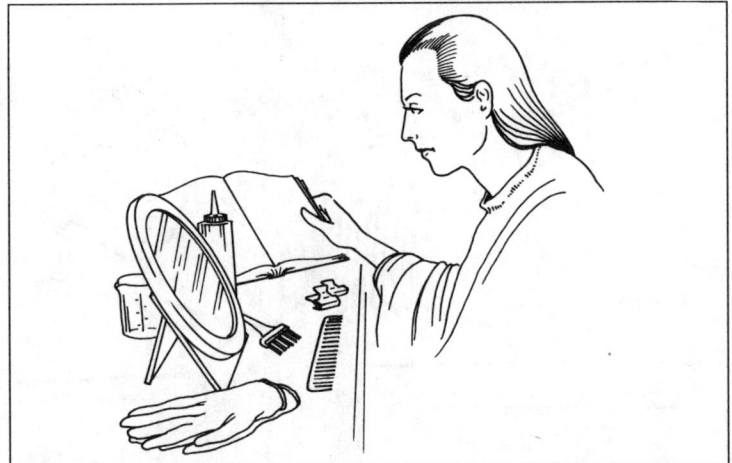

Setting Up To Color Your Hair At Home

The ideal environment for coloring your hair at home is a combination of daylight and incandescent light. Overhead lighting such as track lights or flood lights are also good. Fluorescent lighting makes hair colors and skin tones look drab because they do not show the warm pigments. This means that even though a hair color might have a gold or red tone, the cool fluorescent light will not show that tone. The walls of the room should be a flat white (not shiny) or a soft pastel color such as a very light grey. The area should be warm and draft free. Next, you should have two mirrors set

Getting Started

up: one mirror in front of you and one mirror behind you, with one of these mirrors being movable. With two mirrors, you will be able to see yourself from every angle.

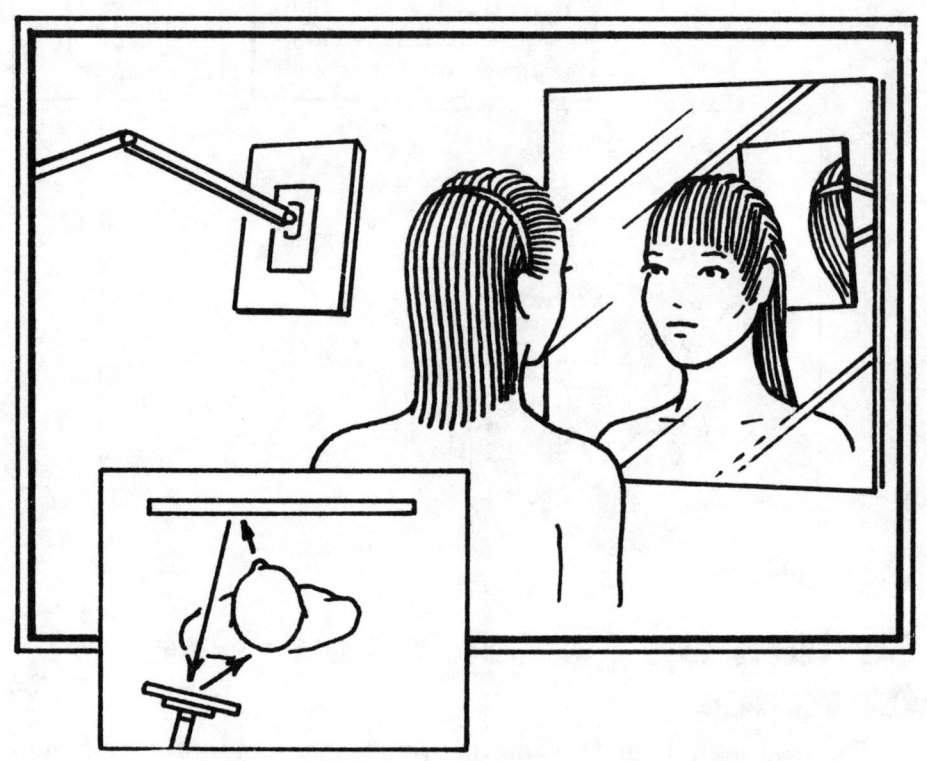

Getting Started

Hair Coloring Accessories

- Shower hose attachable to faucet
- Rubber gloves (buy the ones that are used in beauty salons because they fit better than the ones supplied in the coloring kit)
- Glass or porcelain bowl (the size of a soup bowl)
- Tint brush
- Plastic cape (You can make one from a large garbage bag by cutting an opening for the head and two slits for the arms)
- Applicator bottle
- Glass measuring cup
- Streaking cap with a crochet needle (for strand tests)
- Wide-tooth comb (not metal)
- Four plastic clips that have "teeth" (Jaw-clips used in beauty salons)
- Dark towel
- White towel
- Vaseline
- Shower cap
- Creme rinse
- Protein conditioner
- Shampoo

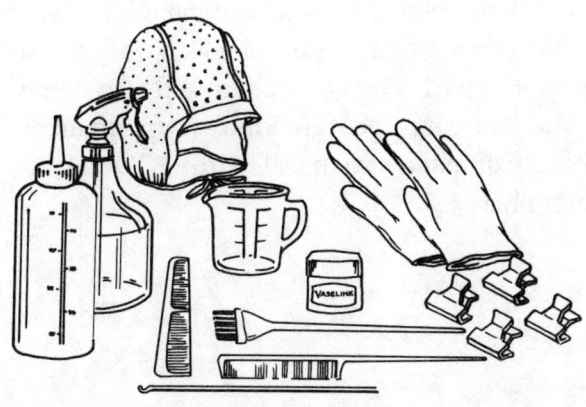

Getting Started

Buying Hair Color In The Drugstore

By the time you are ready to buy your hair color in the drugstore, you should have decided what type of hair color you will need to buy. (See: "Types of Hair Color: To What Extent They Can Change Your Natural Hair Color" on page 24) You should also know the shade and tone that will suit you based on your color-type. (See: "Know Your Color-Type" on page 16)

Hair color products in the drugstore are usually grouped separately according to category. For instance, different brands of semi-permanent rinses are grouped together. It may nevertheless be difficult to distinguish between the different types of hair color. It may be confusing to understand the terminology used on the products as well as the way they are advertised. However, the most important thing you will need to know is if a hair color is a permanent hair color, semi-permanent, etc.

Before you buy a hair color, read the front, back and sides of the bottle or coloring kit. A single bottle means that it is a temporary or semi-permanent color (non-permanent). Permanent and semi-permanent long-lasting hair coloring kits (no ammonia) contain two bottles, consisting of the developer and the hair color. (The kit might also include shampoo and conditioner). A hair lightener kit (bleach) either in oil or creme has three parts, consisting of the bleach, the developer and a little package containing the activator. When you are looking for your shade, you will find that the name of the hair color makes no sense at all. In this case, you will have to look for the generic name of the shade. Verify the shade of the hair color with the color chart. The color chart will also help you choose your hair color. (Make sure it is the right kind - for permanent - or semi-permanent hair color.) Companies such as Clairol, L'Oréal, etc. provide drugstores with color charts.

Getting Started

Which Brand Of Hair Color Should You Buy?

The type of hair color you need in order to achieve the color you want is the most important criteria when buying your hair color in the drugstore. (See: "Selecting And Applying Hair Color" on page 24). Before considering what brand of hair color to buy, you should consider if you need a permanent hair color, a bleach, a semi-permanent hair color or a temporary hair color.

There are several brands of hair coloring products on the market such as Clairol, L'Oréal, Revlon, Max Factor, etc. all of which are considered to be of good quality. These manufacturers also produce "professional" hair coloring products for salons. The basic difference between the products sold in drugstores and the ones that are sold to beauty salons is in the packaging. Although there are several manufacturers of hair coloring products, they all use the same basic technology for making hair color. The only difference may be a personal preference for one manufacturer as opposed to another. It is best to get used to one brand and stay with it. This is exactly what good hair colorists do. Should you like your hair color one level lighter or darker, cooler or warmer, by staying with the same brand, you will know exactly what shade suits you. It is a good idea to keep records of when you colored your hair, and what shade or shades you used (if you custom mix your color). Again, this is what professional hair colorists do. This is helpful if you want to use the same color again or want to change it.

Selecting The Right Color

Why It Is Important To Know The Color Level Of Your Hair Before Coloring Your Hair.

The first step to successfully coloring your hair is knowing the color level of your natural hair color before you apply any hair color to your hair. A color level is the degree of lightness or darkness of a hair color indicated by numbers on the color chart. See: "Chart of Hair Color Levels and Tones" on page 16. The resulting color will depend on your natural hair color or your base color. Knowing the shade of your natural hair color is important for two reasons. First, it will determine what is technically possible. Let's assume you want to be a very light blonde. You have seen the commercials on TV and ads in magazines which tell you that all you have to do is buy a "Shampoo-In Hair Color" in a light blonde (permanent hair color shade), put it on your hair and in 25 minutes you will be a real blonde. The result? A very brassy hair color that doesn't resemble a light blonde shade at all. Why did this happen? Because you put a "Very Light Blonde" shade on your medium brown hair. Had you known how dark your hair really was and had you known your hair was a meduim brown, you would surely not have chosen such a light shade, since the chart on the hair coloring kit indicates that the very light blonde color is only suitable for natural hair colors not darker than dark blonde. These subtle differences in shades significantly influence the outcome. Technically it is not possible to achieve a very light blonde shade when starting out with such a dark base color. Here is another example: You are thinking of putting a henna into your hair. The way you see it is that your natural hair color looks brownish and sometimes in the sunlight it looks like you have reddish highlights. An auburn henna would probably look great, right? Wrong. The resulting color is dark and red and doesn't look like you at all. Had you known that your natural color was medium ash blonde, you would never have chosen that shade. Auburn which is on a level 3 is much darker than medium ash blonde which is on a level 6. See: "Chart of Hair Color Levels and Tones" on page 16. Also if you knew that a red tone didn't suit you, you wouldn't have chosen it which points to the second reason why it is so important to know your natural hair color before you

Selecting The Right Color

choose your new hair color. **Your natural hair color serves as your guide for choosing the right shade and tone.** (See: "Know Your Color-Type: Choosing The Color That Suits You" on page 16.)

Now let's see what you have to do to determine the color level of your hair.

How You Can Determine Your Hair Color Level

Step 1: Your hair should be clean and dry. Wet and oily hair always appears darker. You will need a color chart with swatches of all the color levels. It is best to do this in a drugstore that has color charts. You may also want to bring along a friend to assist you.

Step 2: Part your hair on top or on the side of your head.

Step 3: Hold it apart with both hands. Raise the hair a little by pushing it up with your hands against your head.

Step 4: Have the other person hold a hair swatch form the color chart alongside your hair, close to your scalp. Compare different shades until you find the one that matches your own.

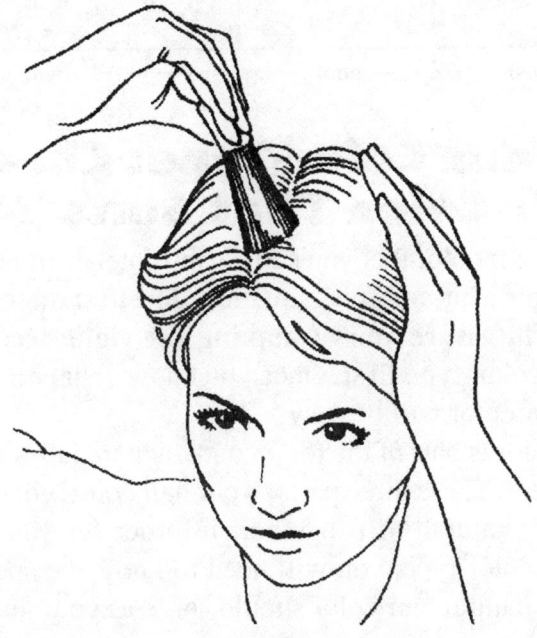

Selecting The Right Color

Chart of Hair Color Levels and Tones

Level	Basic Shades	Ash Shades	Gold and Red Shades	
8	Very Light Blonde	Very Light Ash Blonde	Extra Light Golden Blonde	--- ---
7	Light Blonde	Light Ash Blonde	Light Golden Blonde	Strawberry Blonde
6	Medium Blonde	Medium Ash Blonde	Medium Golden Blonde	Copper
5	Dark Blonde	Dark Ash Blonde	Dark Golden Blonde	Mahogany
4	Light Brown	Light Ash Brown	Light Golden Brown	Chestnut
3	Medium Brown	Medium Ash Brown	Medium Warm Brown	Auburn
2	Dark Brown	--- ---	--- ---	Burgundy
1	Black	---	---	---

|——basic——|——cool——|——warm——|

Know Your Color-Type: Choosing The Hair Color That Suits You

Choosing a hair color that you can be absolutely certain will suit you is for many people a hit-and-miss situation. **The best method to use, the method that will assure you of making the right decision involves knowing your color-type first.** Once you know your color-type, choosing the right hair color will be easy.

Your hair color is part of the total you which includes your skin tone and your eye color. These three parts - your hair color, your skin tone and your eye color - naturally fit together. In order for you to be able to determine your color-type, you will need to know the specific color of your hair. Your natural hair color should serve as your guide. It may be

Selecting The Right Color

helpful at this point to re-read the section on "Why It Is Important To Know The Color Level of Your Hair Before Coloring Your Hair" on page 14 as well as the chart on "Hair Color Levels and Tones" on page 16. As each color-type is described, you will recognize which type applies to you. At the same time you will learn which hair color change would be most flattering for you. Follow these guidelines and your hair color choice will never again be left to chance.

We all fall into two major color-types. But you may be asking yourself "what is a color-type"? People who have light red hair, dark red hair, reddish brown and gold blonde hair represent a "warm" color-type (Autumn and Spring). Red and gold hair pigments are most visible in these hair colors. At the same time, the skin tone and eye color match the "warm" hair color of these color-types. The second group consists of people whose hair is black, mousey brown, mousey blonde, dirty blonde (ash blonde) and in rare cases platinum blonde. Although these people also have some red or gold pigments in their hair, the majority of the pigments are ash or cool (no visible red or gold). These hair colors are described as "cool" and belong to the "cool" color-type (Winter and Summer).

Your color-type should be your guide when choosing a hair color. Simply stated, if you are a "warm" color-type, you should choose a warm tone and if you are a "cool" color-type, you should choose a cool tone. (See Color-Chart on page 16) For example, you would be making a hair coloring error if you were to color your red hair platinum blonde, tint your white hair strawberry blonde (even though your original hair color was a light ash brown) or put reddish-gold highlights into your ash blonde hair. In each case, you would be using a color tone suited for the opposite color-type. The only way you could achieve congruency in these cases would be to change your skin tone and eye color. Let's be more specific now and describe in detail the "warm" and "cool" color-types. Actually each color-type consists of two sub-types - "strong" and "soft".

> In short this is the formula to follow when choosing your hair color: Determining your natural hair color → tells you your color-type → which tells you what shade and tone of hair color to choose.

Selecting The Right Color

What Color-Type Are You?
Guidelines For Determining Your Color-Type.

The Strong-Cool Color-Type (Winter)

Cool is a term that is used to describe a color tone which lacks warmth. It is also described as drab or ash. If you fall into this sub-type, your natural hair color will be black, dark brown, medium brown, light ash brown or platinum blonde. There is no red or gold visible in these colors unless the sun or light hits the hair at a certain angle. With the exception of white and light blonde hair, every hair color has some warm pigments. Your eyes are either dark brown, brown, green, light blue, bluish violet or green with white flecks and a grey rim around the edge of the iris. The iris which is in strong contrast to the white of the eye is especially characteristic of this strong-cool color-type. Diana Ross, Elizabeth Taylor, Sean Connery and Al Pacino are typical examples of the strong-cool color-type.

The Right Color Changes

As previously mentioned, the two main reasons we want to color our hair is either to cover white/grey hair or to make a hair color more interesting. If you want to color white/grey hair, then you will need to remember the color of your hair before it turned white (refer to the color chart swatches in the drug store). If you think the dark hair that is mixed in with your white hair is black, the first time you color your hair you should use a medium brown or light brown shade in order to make sure that the new color is not too dark. The same principle applies when you color hair that is completely white. However, if you find that you look better in a darker shade, then use a darker color the next time you color your hair.

You have probably heard people say that as a person gets older their hair color looks better lighter because of changes in skin tone. This opinion probably comes from the fact that when your hair turns grey/white, it becomes almost lifeless, significantly affecting the skin tone. No matter how striking white/grey or salt and pepper hair looks by itself, it

Selecting The Right Color

drains the color from the face because it lacks pigment. It is the color (pigments) in hair that gives life and expression to hair and skin. Always remember to stay within your color-type. Lightening a hair color is usually not intended for the strong-cool color-types whose hair colors are dark. These are your natural hair colors and match your skin tone. When strong- cool color-types become lighter, they take on the hair color of a different color-type. They won't look as great as they would if they were to stay within their own color-type.

Medium and light brown hair should only have a few highlights. The tone should of course be cool, such as a very light beige. Silver highlights tend to look like white hair. (See: "How to Highlight Your Hair" on page 61). Dark brown and medium brown hair can be colored in tones such as black cherry, plum, cyclamen or burgundy. These tones have a violet blue base which is cool and therefore suited to this color-type. (See: "A Little Bit of Color Theory" on page 74). If you want to change your hair color to blonde, it would have to be to a platinum blonde. However this would require bleaching and a toner every four weeks on the re-growth, making it both time consuming as well as extremely hard on your hair. (See: "The Two-Step Method For Coloring Your Hair Light Blonde" on page 66).

The Wrong Color Changes:
Gold or red highlights, strawberry reds, copper, mahogany, chestnut, gold-blonde and ash blondes.

Selecting The Right Color

The Soft-Cool Color-Type (Summer)

The other "cool" color-type is the "soft"-cool color-type which includes hair colors that most people would describe as mousey or dirty blonde (ash tones). Like the pigments in the "strong"-cool color-type, the cool pigments in this color-type are more visible. Unlike the hair colors constituting the strong-cool color-type, the colors in this group are lighter and can be seen in dark ash blonde, medium ash blonde (these two shades often are mistakenly referred to as "brown") and light ash blonde. Ash is the hair color term for the absence of visible red or gold pigments. If you are a soft-cool color-type, the color of your eyes is either a soft warm brown, blue, green grey, or hazel with a bit of blue and green. Candice Bergen, Farah Fawcett, Linda Evans, Kevin Costner, Ryan O'Neil and Mats Wilander are examples of the soft-cool color-type.

The Right Color Changes

The soft-cool color-type is the color-type that is best suited for streaks/highlights. Your streaks/highlights should be very light (bleached to a pale yellow) and your type can have a lot of them. (See: "How To Highlight Your Hair" on page 61). If your hair is almost white, you can have streaks. The white strands that are bleached will take on a very light blonde tone when they blend in with the rest of the hair, making this color look absolutely striking. (The reason why white hair turns very light blonde when bleached is because hair is 97% keratin-protein). If your hair is completely white, you can tint your hair back to its original color and then add highlights.

The Wrong Color Changes:

You would be moving into the wrong color-type if you were to change your hair to a darker color or if you were to choose a color with red or gold tones in it.

Selecting The Right Color

The Strong-Warm Color-Type (Autumn)

Warm is the term used to describe a hair color that has a lot of red and gold pigments, creating a warm tone. In this color-type, your hair color is either red, strawberry blonde, light golden brown, dark auburn, medium auburn and in a few cases black. Your eyes are either clear green, steel blue, green with golden flecks or warm brown. Many people with this color type have freckles. Katherine Hepburn, Shirley McLaine, Ann Margaret and Robin Williams are examples of this color-type.

The Right Color Changes

The most important point to remember when coloring your hair is to use a hair color in a warm tone (But not too light). You can add warm tone highlights such as gold and red (See: "How To Highlight Your Hair" on page 61). Henna is ideally suited for this color-type. See: "Henna" on page 39. For coloring hair that is mostly white, See: "Tinting White/Grey Hair Red" on page 60.

The Wrong Color Changes:

Avoid ash tones, black (unless you are one of the few in this color-type who have black hair), burgundy and black cherry (these tones are cool). Also unsuited are a lot of light highlights which will make your hair color appear too light. The cool tone of the streaks will clash with the warm tone of your hair.

Selecting The Right Color

The Soft-Warm Color-Type (Spring)

If you fall into this category, your hair color is either golden blonde, strawberry blonde, chestnut, medium warm blonde, light copper, honey blonde or light golden brown. The color of your eyes is clear blue, aqua, hazel with green in it, or green with gold in it. Typical examples of this color-type are Debbie Reynolds, Glenn Close, Julie Andrews and Robert Redford.

The Right Color Changes

Color your hair in a warm tone. If you want to color white hair, then use the color of the hair that has not yet turned white as your guideline for choosing a hair color. If your hair is no more than 30% white, Henna will make it look natural. For completely white hair, the best type of hair color is a permanent hair color in a warm tone. You could also put golden highlights into your hair. See: "How to Highlight Your Hair" on page 61.

The Wrong Color Changes:
Don't color your hair black, dark or medium auburn, brown, ash blonde, burgundy or streak it very light.

Selecting The Right Color

The Four Color-Types and How Their Hair Can Be Colored

Natural Hair Color of the Four Color-Types	Use
Strong-Cool: Black Dark Brown Medium Brown Light Brown Platinum Blonde (rare) White/Grey/Salt & Pepper	• Semi-permanent hair color in tones such as burgundy and plum • Henna in shades of brown and natural to give luster to your hair • Use either a long-lasting semi-permanent hair color or permanent hair color matching the level of your own hair color • Lowlighting
Soft-Cool: Very Light Ash Brown Light Ash Blonde Medium Ash Blonde Dark Ash Brown White/Grey	• Streaks • Permanent hair color matching your own ash blonde; then streak • Streak only
Strong-Warm: Warm Brown Auburn Mahogany Red White/Grey	• Use Henna in warm tones to intensify your hair color • Add gold, reddish highlights • Use a semi-permanent rinse in warm tones
Soft-Warm: Honey Blonde Light Gold Blonde Strawberry Blonde Chestnut White/Grey	• Use Henna in warm tones to intensify your hair color • Use a semi-permanent rinse in warm tones • Add gold highlights • For more than 30% grey hair, use permanent hair color in warm tones

Selecting And Applying Hair Color

Hair colors are often named and advertised in a way that makes it hard to know which category they fall into. Drugstore shelves are full of all kinds of hair coloring products. It can be very confusing if you don't know what you are looking for.

Types Of Hair Colors: To What Extent They Can Change Your Natural Hair Color.

Temporary Color Rinse	Semi-Permanent Color Rinse I	Semi-Permanent Color Rinse II	Permanent Hair Color	Bleach
1	2	3	4	5
The least change Does not cover white hair	Hardly covers white hair Cannot make hair lighter	Covers white hair well but only in dark shades Cannot make hair lighter	Covers white hair well Can lighten and color your hair at the same time	The most change Removes color

Number 1 represents the least color change whereas number 5 represents the most color change you can achieve with this particular type of hair color. What will these products do for your hair? Should you experiment and see what it looks like in your hair? Definitely not! The purpose of this book is to take the guesswork out of coloring your hair. Each type of hair color has a specific use as well as advantages and disadvantages. Once you know what each one does, you will be in the position to decide what type you want to use on your hair and why.

Selecting And Applying Hair Color

Selecting Between Temporary Rinses, Semi-Permanent Rinses Permanent Hair Color And Bleach

(a) Hair color that washes out of your hair is called a temporary and semi-permanent rinse.

(b) Hair color that does not wash out of your hair is called a permanent hair color. (A bleach is designed to remove pigments from your hair.)

Temporary Rinse

The temporary rinse is a diluted water color, capable of producing very little change in the color of your hair. It lasts for only one shampoo, thereby the term "temporary".

When To Use A Temporary Rinse

a) The most practical use for a temporary rinse is to soften the harshness of white/grey hair by giving it a silver, steel grey or silver blue tone.

Natural Hair Color	Hair Colors to Use i.e. Fanci-full rinse by Roux
• White Hair - 90 to 100% white	White Minx, Silver Lining
• Grey Hair - 60% white - 40% dark	Platinum Plus, True Steel
• Salt & Pepper Hair - 40% white - 60% dark	Black Rage

b) The above mentioned tones can also be used to neutralize yellow in white hair. (See: "A Little Bit of Color Theory" on page 74).

c) Tones such as White Minx, Demure Mist, Platinum Plus and Bashful Blonde will also neutralize the yellow in pale yellow bleached hair.

NOTE:
Please follow the instructions on how to apply a temporary rinse with cotton wool. Otherwise the color will remain mostly in the ends.

Selecting and Applying Hair Color

What it cannot be used for:
A temporary hair color cannot be used to cover white hair, make a color lighter or create any depth in color.

How long will a temporary rinse last?
The color disappears after one shampoo and will come off on pillows and collars.

Selecting and Applying Hair Color

How To Apply A Temporary Rinse

You will need a plastic cape, rubber gloves, two mirrors of which one is movable (one in the front and one in the back), a little glass bowl, cottonwool, a dark towel and a tail comb.

Shampoo, towel dry your hair and apply a creme rinse.

There are two ways to apply a temporary rinse. One way consists of applying the rinse directly from the bottle into your hair while gently working it into your hair. This method is suitable for hair colors that are not light blonde or pale yellow blonde.

The second method is used for bleached hair.

Step 1: Pour one ounce of rinse into a little glass bowl. Using a tail comb, divide your hair making a part on top of your head, starting at the middle of your forehead and working your way down to the crown. Dip a piece of cottonwool into the rinse, squeezing some of the liquid out. Using the cottonwool, apply the rinse on your hair but only from the roots to the middle of your hair, bypassing the ends. Having the consistency of water, the rinse will naturally saturate the ends when the hair is combed through. Because the ends of bleached hair are always more porous, they absorb more of the color than the rest of the hair. If you also apply the rinse directly on the ends, you will end up with two different shades - the roots and the middle of your hair will be yellow whereas the ends will be silvery.

Step 2: Make a horizontal part one inch below the first one. Using cottonwool, apply the rinse up to the middle of the hair again bypassing the ends. Continue in this way until you have covered both sides. Now make a horizontal part on the back of the crown. Continue making one inch wide parts and applying the rinse. When you have reached the nape, comb your hair through.

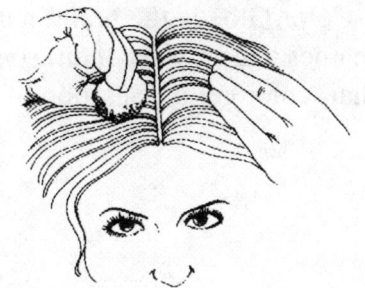

27

Selecting And Applying Hair Color

Brand names of temporary rinses:
- Fanci-full Rinse (Roux)
- Instant Beauté (Clairol)
- Coloral (L'Oréal)

Other Temporary Colors

These temporary colors come in "fantasy" colors such as gold, silver, blue, pink, green, etc. They also come in spray cans and are sprayed on just like spray paint. Their coloring agent is food coloring. The other "fantasy" temporary hair color comes in gel form.

How To Spray Color Your Hair
- Spray the color on your finished hairstyle.
- Hold a piece of cardboard behind you so as not to spray anything else or as a way of keeping colors separate when using more than one color. If your hair becomes wet, the color will come off on your clothes.

NOTE: If your hair is bleached, it will be difficult to shampoo the color out of your hair.

How To Apply Gel "Fantasy" Temporary Colors
- Use the gel on your finished hairstyle.
- Take an 8 inch long string and saturate it in the gel.

Now hold it firmly on each end and press it lightly on your hair. You can create a design this way. This technique works best on smooth hairstyles. "Color Glo" is the brand name of a temporary hair color spray. Brand names will vary depending on where you live. An example of a temporary hair color gel is "Sassoon".

Selecting And Applying Hair Color

The Color Stick

The color stick also falls into the category of a temporary hair color. It is used on grey roots, around the hair line and in between touch-ups. These sticks come in several colors, ranging from medium blonde to black. The color washes out after one shampoo.

How to Apply a Color Stick

Dampen the color stick and color the new growth, using a shade that matches your own.

Brand Name: Color Stick by Roux

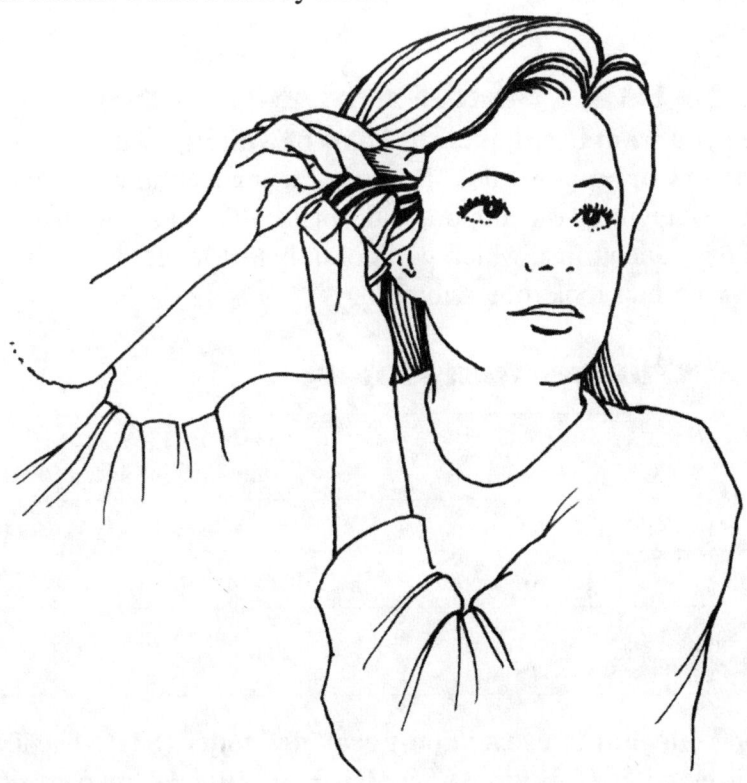

Selecting And Applying Hair Color

Semi-Permanent Hair Color
Category I

The semi-permanent hair color attaches itself to the outside of the hair, coating the hair with color. After about six shampoos, the color will wash out. It contains no peroxide (developer) and no ammonia. When you buy this type of color in the drugstore, the box will contain one bottle which you can apply directly on your hair.

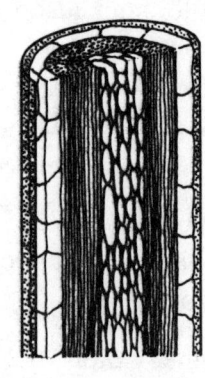

semi-permanent color on the cuticle ←

(cross section of of a hair)

When to Use a Semi-Permanent Rinse

a) **When you want to enhance the color of white/grey hair by giving it a silvery or smokey look.** Instead of using a temporary rinse that washes out with one shampoo, you can use the following shades of a semi-permanent rinse which will not only last longer but will also make your hair look more vibrant.

How to Choose Your Color

Hair Color	Color To Use
	(for example Silk & Silver - Clairol)
White Hair - 90% to 100% white	Silver White, Silvery Pearl
Grey Hair - 60% white - 40% dark	Silver Mist, Silvery Smoke
Salt & Pepper Hair - 40% white - 60% dark	Silvery Slate

b) **When you want to use a "non-peroxide" toner** (See: "The Two-Step Method For Coloring Your Hair Light Blonde" on page 66). It can give pale yellow bleached hair a pastel blonde shade. Born Blonde by Clairol is a popular brand.

30

Selecting And Applying Hair Color

c) **When you want to add vibrancy to the hair color of warm color-types.** (See: Know Your Color-Type on page 16). The color you choose should be similar to your own natural hair color. (See: Color Chart on page 16). For example, if your natural hair color is medium brown, you should choose an auburn hair color because it is at the same color level as your own natural hair color. If you choose a shade that is lighter than your own color, there will be no change in your hair color because a semi-permanent rinse is not capable of making hair lighter. In addition to the warm color-types, the strong-cool color-type is also a candidate for a semi-permanent color rinse but in tones of burgundy, wine, black cherry, plum, etc.

Read the information on the box or check the color chart on the instruction sheet to ensure that you know exactly what a particular color is used for and for what natural hair color. For example, Flirt-Gel Hair Blush (Clairol) has the following tones:

Kohl for dark brown or black hair
Raisin for dark brown or black hair
Cassis for dark brown or black hair
Grenadine for medium brown or medium auburn hair
Champagne for light brown or red/auburn hair
Bronze for medium brown to light brown and red/auburn hair

d) **When you want to freshen up a tinted red tone that has faded.**
Tinted (permanent hair color) red hair such as light, medium and dark red tones fade after two weeks. (Red tones always fade the fastest). Instead of re-applying a tint in order to intensify the color, you can simply use a semi-permanent rinse to accentuate the tone in between tints. This strategy has two distinct advantages. First, this type of color lasts longer, because tinted hair is porous and the semi-permanent hair color attaches to it better. Secondly, a semi-permanent rinse cannot damage the hair and therefore keeps it in better condition.

It is important to match the tone of the semi-permanent rinse with your own tinted hair. (See: "How You Can Determine Your Hair

Selecting And Applying Hair Color

Color Level" on page 15). However in this case, the middle section of your hair, that is the section between the roots and the ends, should be used as your guideline. This part of the hair fades the least.

What A Semi-Permanent Rinse Cannot Be Used For

A semi-permanent color cannot change the pigments in your hair and therefore cannot lighten your hair. For example, a semi-permanent color cannot change dark blonde hair to light blonde. This type of color is also not very effective in covering white/grey hair. It is not suited for the soft-cool color-type since colors such as light blonde, medium ash blonde etc. have no effect on the natural hair color of this color-type. (See: "Know Your Color-Type" on page 16).

The following is a list of some of the semi-permanent rinses available.
- Silk & Silver by Clairol
- Avantage by L'Oréal
- Flirt by Clairol
- Zazu by L'Oréal
- Loving Care by Clairol
- Cost: approximately from $5.00 to $7.00

How long will a semi-permanent color last in your hair?

Approximately for six shampoos.

Selecting And Applying Hair Color

How To Apply A

Step 1: ## Semi-Permanent Color

In addition to the shade of the semi-permanent rinse, you should have the following handy: (See: Setting Up to Color Your Hair at Home on page 9).

Two mirrors - in order to see the back and profile of your head, a plastic cape, rubber gloves, a dark colored towel, vaseline,

Step 2: shampoo and creme rinse.

Step 3: Shampoo your hair and towel dry.

Step 4: Put vaseline on the skin around your hairline. Be careful not to get any vaseline on your hair because the color will not take.

Not being concerned about a re-growth (roots), you can apply the color over your entire hair. Starting at the crown of your head, squeeze the color on your hair while working it into your hair, making sure that every strand is covered with the rinse. Put on a shower cap or a plastic cap and wait 30 minutes (depending on the product instructions). What would happen if you left the rinse on longer than 30 minutes? Not much. After the required time has elapsed, the color will not change. However it may be more difficult to wash off your skin if you forgot to apply vaseline on the skin around the hairline. What you can do in this case is to use a skin stain remover and/or apply a facial cream on the stained areas, leaving them on for several hours. What happens if you shampoo the rinse out before the recommended processing time? The color will not have had enough time to attach itself to the hair and you will not get the desired result.

Selecting And Applying Hair Color

Choosing The Right Semi-Permanent Hair Color Tone For Your Color-Type

Category I

This chart can be used by people who have no grey hair as well as by those who have up to 30% grey hair.

Color-Type	Recommended Hair Color to Use	Resulting Hair Color on Grey Hair
Soft-Warm	Gold Blonde Strawberry Blonde	Gold Gold
Strong-Warm	Bronze Champagne Grenadine Golden Brown Golden Copper Brown Copper Auburn	Gold Gold Red Reddish Light Gold Brown Red/Copper Dark Reddish
Soft-Cool	—	—
Strong-Cool	Dark Ash Brown Black Medium Ash Brown Light Ash Brown Burgundy Brown Black Cherry	Light Brown Black Gold Brown Gold Burgundy Dark Cherry

Selecting And Applying Hair Color

Category II

This type of hair color is a long-lasting semi-permanent hair color. It is a cross between a permanent hair color and a semi-permanent rinse. It has no ammonia but requires a developer. Instead of only coating the hair with color, a long-lasting semi-permanent hair color slightly penetrates the hair cuticle making the color last longer than the semi-permanent rinse. This type of hair color is ideal for the strong-cool color-type because it never becomes brassy.

When to use a long-lasting semi-permanent rinse

When you want to color white/grey hair dark and don't want to use a permanent hair color (tint). Although long-lasting semi-permanent rinse shades range from black to ash blonde, only the darker shades are really effective in covering white hair.

Choosing the Right Long-Lasting Semi-Permanent Rinse Tone

Color-Type	Recommended Hair Color To Use
Soft-Warm	—
Strong-Warm	Auburn
Soft-Cool	—
Strong-Cool	Black Dark Ash Brown Medium Ash Brown Burgundy

BRAND NAMES:
- Clairesse by Clairol
- Sheer Color Gloss by Clairol

Cost: Approximately from $5.00 to $7.00

Selecting And Applying Hair Color

What a long-lasting semi-permanent hair color cannot be used for:
- It cannot lighten a natural hair color.
- It is not suitable for the soft-warm or the soft-cool color types.

Brand names:
- Sheer Color Gloss by Clairol
- Clairesse by Clairol

How long will a long-lasting semi-permanent color last in your hair?

Generally speaking, a long-lasting semi-permanent color slowly washes out with the darker shades such as black and dark brown lasting several months. If, however, with each application the color is applied over the entire head, it will not wash out.

Selecting And Applying Hair Color

How To Apply A Long-Lasting Semi-Permanent Hair Color

Use this method of application if you are **coloring your hair for the first time.**

Step 1: You will need the following hair coloring accessories: two mirrors, a plastic cape, rubber gloves, a dark colored towel, vaseline, a glass bowl, a tint brush, shampoo, creme rinse and of course your hair color.

Step 2: Put vaseline around your hairline. Brush your hair back. Mix the hair color. Pour the bottle of color into the bottle containing the developer.

Step 3: Squeeze the color on your hair while working it into your hair and making sure that every strand is covered with the rinse. Let it process for 30 minutes. Then rinse, shampoo and condition.

Selecting And Applying Hair Color

Use This Method For Applying The Color On the Re-Growth

To achieve a really natural looking hair color, it is best to apply the long-lasting semi-permanent rinse on the re-growth only.

Step 1: Mix the hair color and developer into a glass bowl. Stir with the tint brush. Brush your unwashed hair back, dampening it with a water bottle.

Step 2: Start by making a part from the middle of the forehead to the crown by sliding the pointy end of the tint brush in a straight line along the scalp toward the crown. Dip the tint brush into the color mixture and paint the color on the re-growth, covering the hair well. Now make another part, sectioning the hair half an inch below the first part and apply the color with a tint brush. Continue to make half inch wide sections until both sides are covered. On the back of your head, make a horizontal section on the crown area, applying the color on the roots only. Continue making horizontal sections in sequence until you reach the nape. Make sure the roots are covered well with color. Leave the color on your hair for 30 minutes. Rinse, shampoo and condition. Discard the mixed, unused formula. (See: "How to Apply a Tint" Technique No. III illustrations on page 47).

NOTE:
Before applying the long-lasting semi-permanent rinse, section a part, about a quarter of an inch in width around the hairline which will not be colored. Slightly wet this section and comb it forward, onto your forehead. Leaving the front uncolored gives hair a more natural look. You can only do this if your hair is no more than 75% white. See: "How to Apply a Tint" and illustration on page 48.

Selecting And Applying Hair Color

Henna

Another type of semi-permanent hair color is a Henna where the color can last longer than six shampoos. In fact if Henna is applied over the entire hair every time it is used, it will hardly wash out. Henna is made from the leaves of a plant found in Asia and Africa. The leaves are dried in the sun and crushed into a powder.

How to Mix and Apply a Henna

Step 1: You should have the following items at your disposal: two mirrors - in order to see the back and profile of your hair, a plastic cap, rubber gloves, a dark colored towel, vaseline, shampoo, creme rinse, a glass (or porcelain) bowl and a tint brush. You will also need hot black coffee, (for mixing the Henna powder - if you don't have coffee, use hot water), the juice of a lemon, (the acidity in the lemon helps the color adhere to the hair) and an egg yolk (to keep the mixture moist and smooth).

Step 2: Empty the Henna into a heavy glass or porcelain bowl (a heavy bowl prevents sliding). Add the hot coffee to the powder and using the tint brush stir the mixture until it turns into a creamy paste. Now add the egg yolk and lemon juice, mixing all the ingredients together.

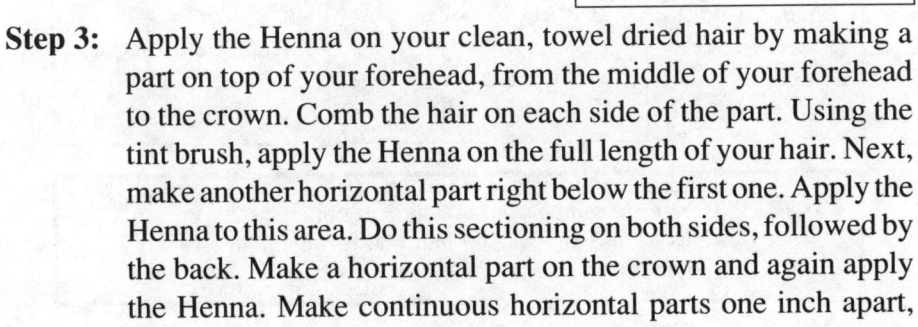

Step 3: Apply the Henna on your clean, towel dried hair by making a part on top of your forehead, from the middle of your forehead to the crown. Comb the hair on each side of the part. Using the tint brush, apply the Henna on the full length of your hair. Next, make another horizontal part right below the first one. Apply the Henna to this area. Do this sectioning on both sides, followed by the back. Make a horizontal part on the crown and again apply the Henna. Make continuous horizontal parts one inch apart,

Selecting And Applying Hair Color

applying the Henna each time, until you reach the nape. (Only if you have very short hair do you not need to section your hair. Otherwise, sectioning helps to ensure even coverage). If you have a regrowth, only apply the Henna to the root area. Put a plastic cap or shower cap over your hair. Process for the time indicated in the instructions. Rinse, shampoo and apply a creme rinse.

Cost: Approximately from $5.00 to $7.00

Choosing The Right Henna Tone For Your Color-Type

This chart can be used by people who have no grey hair as well as by those who have up to 30% grey hair.

Color-Type	Recommended Hair Color To Use	Resulting Hair Color On Grey Hair
Soft-Warm	Wheat Blonde	Gold
	Buttercup	Gold
	Blonde	Gold
	Apricot Blonde	Gold
Strong-Warm	Red Sunset	Red
	Mahogany	Red
	Gold Brown	Dark Gold
	Chestnut	Gold
Soft-Cool	Natural	—
Strong-Cool	Dark Brown	Light Gold Brown
	Brown	Light Gold Brown
	Black	Brown
	Burgundy	Dark Red

NOTE
- Natural can be used on any hair color.
- Don't use a Henna on hair that is more than 30% grey.
- Don't use a Henna on bleached hair.

Selecting And Applying Hair Color

Permanent Hair Color (Tint)

This type of hair color has the greatest versatility and the best color selection. Permanent hair colors change the pigments in your hair, making them impossible to wash out. Your natural hair color will become visible after a few weeks at which time you can tint the re-growth. The distinguishing feature of permanent hair colors is that they can make your hair lighter while coloring it at the same time. They also allow for custom mixing your hair color - mixing more than one shade. (See "Customizing Your Hair Color" on page 72).

When you buy your hair coloring kit, you will notice that the package includes a bottle that contains the color as well as a bottle that contains the developer. The two need to be mixed together before applying the solution. Once the color is mixed, its effectiveness lasts for one hour. Therefore any remaining mixed formula should be discarded after one hour.

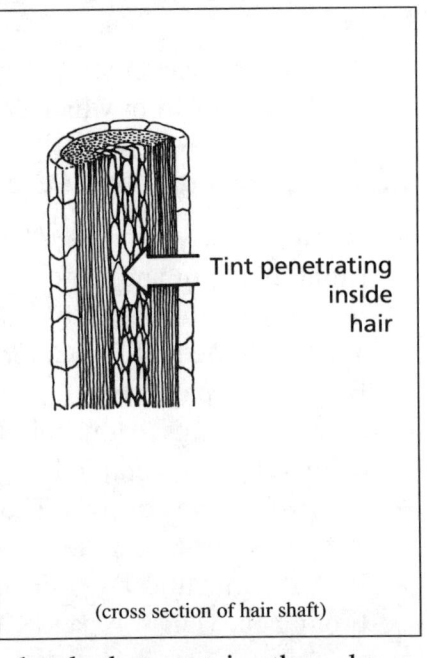

Tint penetrating inside hair

(cross section of hair shaft)

NOTE :
1. Test your tint first to avoid allergic reactions.
2. Test your new hair color first. See "Testing For Allergic Reactions" and "How To Test Your New Hair Color".

When To Use A Permanent Hair Color

- When you want to color your white/grey hair.
- It covers white hair very well - from black to a very light blonde.
- When you want to lighten, highlight your natural hair color.
- It can lighten your natural hair color up to 3 levels.
- It can give light bleached hair a pastel blonde color.

Selecting And Applying Hair Color

How long will a permanent color last in your hair?

A permanent hair color does not wash out. After four weeks, there will be a re-growth of 1 cm which can be tinted.

What you cannot use it for

- A tint cannot lighten your hair from brown (light, medium and dark brown) to a very light blonde or pastel blonde. (See: "The Two-Step Method For Coloring Your Hair Blonde" on page 66).
- It cannot be used on hair that has been colored with a metallic hair color solution such as Grecian Formula. The metallic color has to be removed first. (See: "How to Remove Metallic Dyes-Grecian Formula-From Your Hair" on page 90).

NOTE:
A tint cannot be used to lighten the color of already tinted hair. It can only lighten an untinted, natural hair color. An artificial pigment cannot lighten another artificial pigment.

Selecting And Applying Hair Color

How To Apply A Tint

Get ready to color your hair by going over the list of accessories suggested in the section on "Setting Up to Color Your Hair at Home" on page 9. There are three different techniques for correctly applying a tint. However, prior to using any of these techniques you should not shampoo your hair for at least one day. This allows for the natural oils to be present in the hair and scalp.

- Put vaseline around your hairline.

Technique Number I
This technique is used when applying a tint with an applicator bottle on very short hair or on hair that is being colored for the first time.

Technique Number II
This technique is used when applying a tint with an applicator bottle on a re-growth of one cm but not on the ends.

Technique Number III
This technique is used when applying a tint with a tint brush on a re-growth of more than one cm but not on the ends.

Technique Number I

Step 1: Take the two bottles out of the hair coloring kit and mix the color and the developer in the applicator bottle.

Step 2: Squeeze the mixture on your hair, beginning at the crown and then over the rest of your hair, using one hand to work the color into your hair. Avoid rubbing it into your scalp as it will irritate it. Work the color into a lather making sure to thoroughly cover all your hair. Leave the color on your hair for 30 minutes.

Step 3: Rinse thoroughly, shampoo once and apply a protein conditioner.

Selecting And Applying Hair Color

Technique Number II

Using the applicator bottle, apply the color only on the roots. Be careful not to put any tint on the ends. Otherwise you will put tint on top of tint every time you color your hair, drying out your hair unnecessarily. Applying the color only on the roots will also prevent the ends from becoming darker and darker when you use darker shades. Although a permanent hair color fades from one tint to the next, it does not mean that the ends remain faded when using the above mentioned method. In the process of rinsing off the tint, enough color pigments will be absorbed by the ends to restore the depth of color that was missing before.

Exceptions to this method:
a) if you change to another color
b) if you need to make a color correction (See: "How to Correct Undesirable Hair Colors" on page 76)
c) if you want to intensify a red tone.

Step 1: Mix the tint into an applicator bottle.

Step 2: Dampen your hair by spraying it lightly with a plant moisturizing bottle. Brush your hair back.

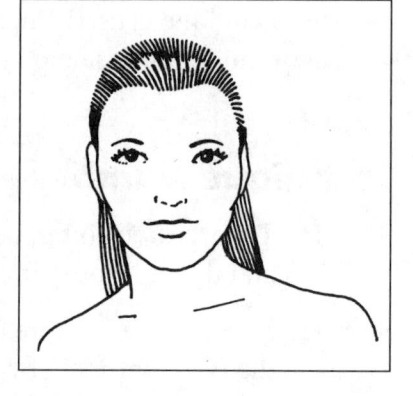

Step 3: Start applying the color by making a part from the middle of your forehead to the crown and sliding the tip of the applicator bottle nozzle along your scalp in a straight line. Hold up one part of the separated section and squeeze the color on the roots from the crown to the hairline. Repeat the same process, parting the hair a half inch below the first part. Continue this process until each side of the head is done.

Selecting And Applying Hair Color

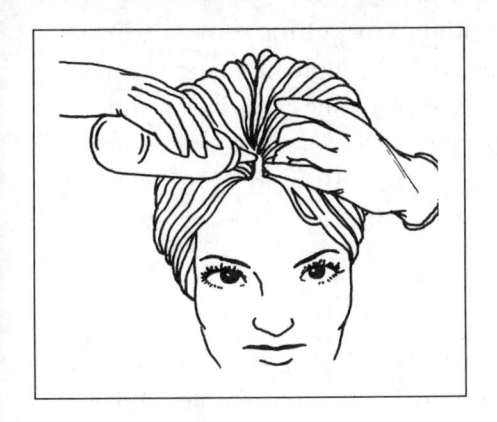

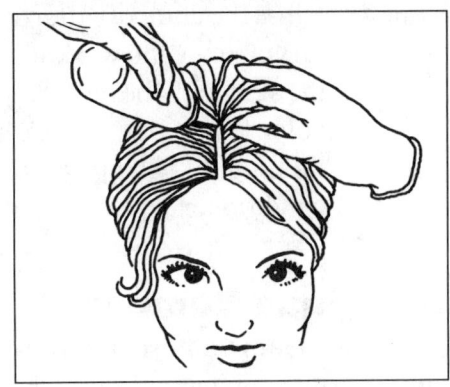

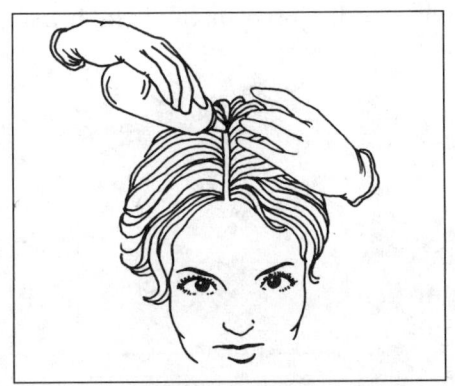

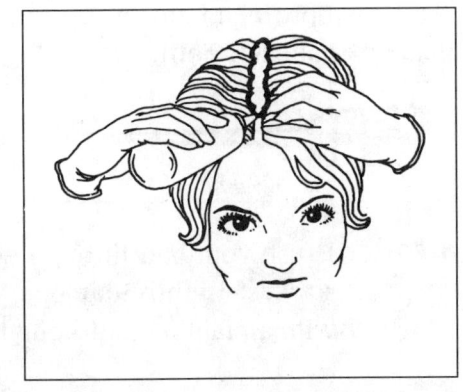

Now comes the back of your head (Since you are working with two mirrors this should not be difficult). Using the nozzle of the applicator bottle, make a horizontal part on the crown on the back of your head. Continue making half inch wide sections from side to side of your head until you reach the nape.

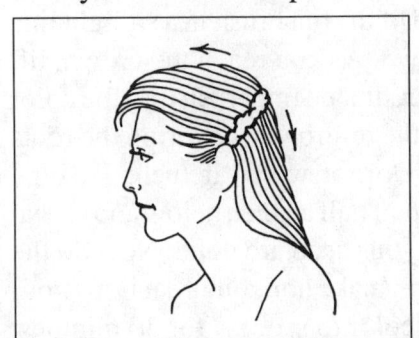

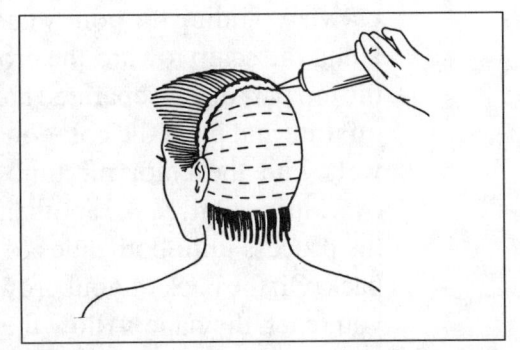

Selecting And Applying Hair Color

Step 4: Rinse the color off after 30 minutes by putting some warm water on your hair and working the color through your hair. Gently rub the skin with the color along your hairline. This will remove the color from your skin. Add more and more water rinsing it out thoroughly. Shampoo once. Towel dry and apply a protein conditioner.

Technique Number III

Why should you use a tint brush? Hair colorists use a tint brush to apply permanent hair colors because it gives them more control. If your roots are more then 1 cm long, you can do a better job by using a tint brush than an applicator bottle.

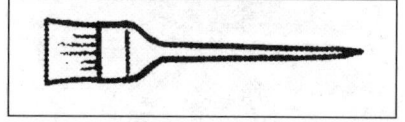

Step 1: Brush your hair through with a few strokes. Lightly dampen your hair with a plant moisturizing bottle.

Step 2: In a glass or porcelain bowl, mix the color and the developer, using the tint brush to blend the mixture.

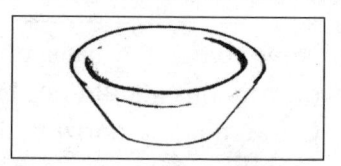

Step 3: Start by making a part from the middle of your forehead to the crown by sliding the pointy end of the tint brush in a straight line along the scalp toward the crown. As you reach the crown, lift the top part of the separated hair, dip the tint brush into the color mixture and paint the color on the re-growth, covering the roots well with the color mixture. Do not worry if there is some overlap in color. Make another part half an inch below and repeat the process until both sides of your head are done. Now do the back. On the back of your crown, make horizontal sections until you reach the nape. Allow the color to process for 30 minutes.

Selecting And Applying Hair Color

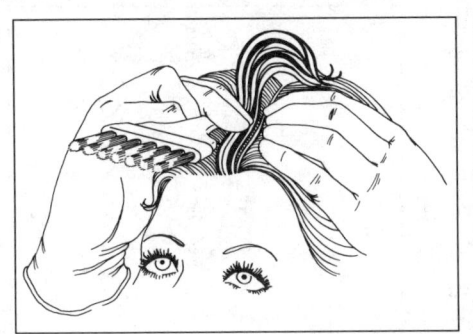

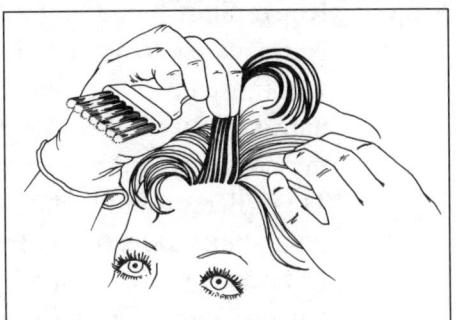

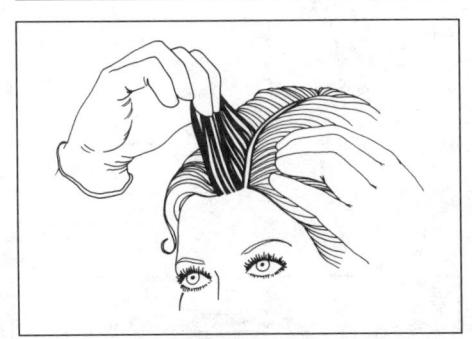

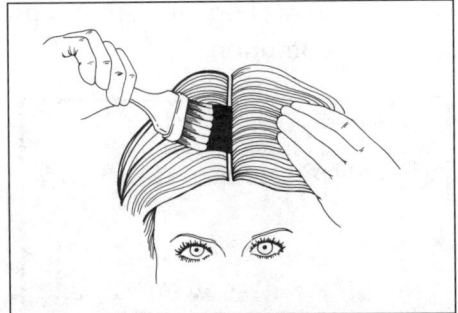

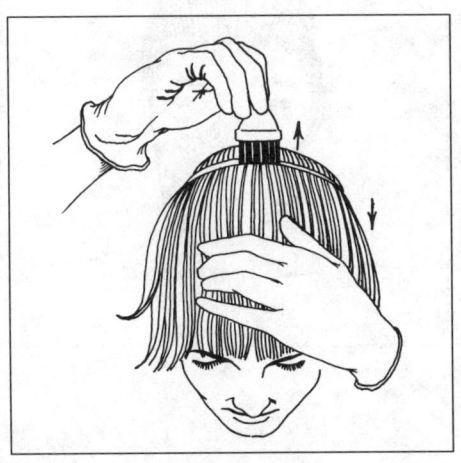

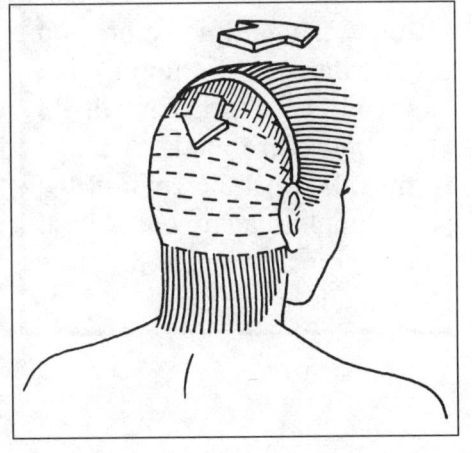

Selecting And Applying Hair Color

Step 4: Rinse. Start by adding a little warm water to your hair and working the color into your hair. Gently rub the skin with the color around the hairline. This will remove the stain from your skin. Add more and more water, rinsing the color mixture out thoroughly. Shampoo once. Towel dry and apply a protein conditioner.

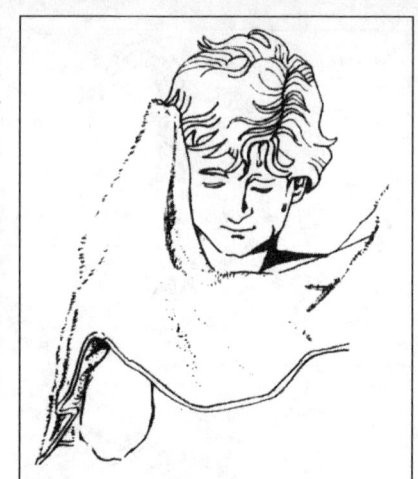

NOTE:
(For hair that is up to 75% white/grey)
If you want to prevent the re-growth from showing around the hairline, leave out the hair around the hairline before you apply the tint. Wet this section of your hair and comb it on to your forehead. Always remember that the color of the tint should match your natural hair color when using this technique.

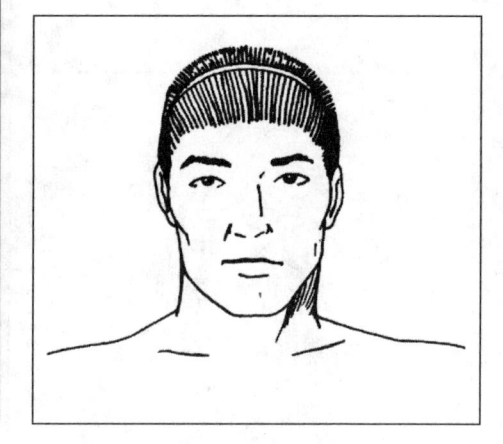

Selecting And Applying Hair Color

Important Points To Remember When Tinting Your Hair

1. Make sure that your own hair color and the color you choose are similar. For example, if your own hair is brown, you should not use a light blonde color. Even if you use a highlighting hair color such as Miss Clairol's Extra Lightening Hair Color, you will still end up with an undesired gold/brassy tone. If you want to change your color to blonde and your own hair color is darker than dark blonde, you will need to use the double-process blonding technique. (See: "The Two-Step Method For Coloring Your Hair Light Blonde" on page 66).

2. If your hair is already tinted but you find the color too dark, you cannot use a tint in a lighter shade in order to lighten your color. An artificial pigment cannot lighten another artificial pigment.

3. Hair color that has been mixed with developer cannot be used after one hour.

4. If the bottle containing the hair color or the developer is left open, it will lose its effect.

5. Hair that is 100% white can be colored with any shade, ranging from black to platinum blonde.

6. Never use a red tone by itself on white hair. Always use a basic hair color (permanent hair color) (see color chart p.16) as part of the formula.

7. Do not use an ash tone on 100% white hair. Always use a basic hair color (permanent hair color) (see color chart p.16) as part of the formula.

8. The color on the first inch of your hair will appear lighter than the color on the rest of your hair. The reason for this is that the light is reflected differently on the newest growth of your hair because the cuticle on this part of the hair lies flat. (See: "The Chemistry of Your Hair" on page 93).

Selecting And Applying Hair Color

9. The best type of hair color to cover white/grey hair is a permanent hair color.

> **NOTE:**
> There is an easy and simple way to put highlights in your hair while at the same time tinting your hair. (Mix the tint and developer from two hair coloring kits to ensure that you have enough hair color for this application).
>
> Every so often it will become necessary to apply the tint not only on the roots but all the way through to the ends when the color has faded to a much lighter shade. Now instead of making it one solid shade, you can leave out strands when applying the color throughout. These strands of course will remain lighter, thus making it look like you have highlights.

How to do this:

Using the pointy end of the tint brush, section the hair and apply the tint on the re-growth (see technique number III on page 46). Allow the color to develop on the roots for 15 minutes. Now you can apply the color to the rest of the hair by again making half inch wide sections and applying the color all the way to the ends but leaving out strands of hair in each section which will not be colored. Wait 15 minutes before rinsing off the color. Then shampoo and apply a conditioner.

Selecting And Applying Hair Color

Metallic Hair Dye

Another type of hair color is a metallic dye, sometimes referred to as a progressive dye. Men who have grey hair often use this type of hair color because it is advertised as a hair coloring product for men even though all hair coloring products are unisex. One well known brand is Grecian Formula. This type of hair color is called a metallic dye because it contains either lead, silver or copper derivatives. The hair coloring liquid is applied directly from the bottle on the hair. With daily or weekly use, white hair turns darker and darker. No color selection is available with this type of hair color. When it has reached the color depth you want, the solution only needs to be applied twice a week in order to be maintained. Although the color does not penetrate the hair, it is hard to shampoo out. You should not have a perm, tint or bleach if your hair is colored with a metallic dye. The chemicals in the metallic dye are not compatible with the chemicals in a tint, bleach, perm, etc. (See: "How to Remove Metallic Hair Color from you Hair" on page 90).

When To Use A Metallic Hair Dye

Today it is no longer necessary to use this type of hair color. It was for many years the accepted hair color for men and mostly marketed for men, stressing a very natural look. Unfortunately this kind of hair color does not look nearly as natural as hair colors marketed for women. As I have mentioned before there is no difference between men's and women's hair and men, of course, can use the same hair colors as women.

Selecting And Applying Hair Color

Bleach (Pre-Lightening)

The function of a hair bleach is to remove the dark pigments from hair, thereby lightening the color.

When should you bleach your hair?
1. When your hair is too dark to achieve a pastel blonde using a tint. (See: Two-Step Method For Coloring Your Hair Blonde on page 66).
2. When making color corrections. (See: "Correcting Undesirable Hair Colors" on page 76).
3. When streaking, highlighting, and frosting. (See: " How To Highlight Your Hair" on page 61).

As hair is bleached, it goes through different color levels. A bleach always produces warm tones. Black hair will go through the following color changes when being bleached to light yellow:

> Level 1: Black to Dark Red Brown (Level 2)
> Level 2: Dark Red Brown to Med. Red Brown (Level 3)
> Level 3: Med. Red Brown to Red (Level 4)
> Level 4: Red to Bronze (Level 5)
> Level 5: Orange to Gold (Level 6)
> Level 6: Gold to Yellow (Level 7)
> Level 7: Yellow to Pale Yellow (Level 8)

You can stop the lightening process at any level simply by rinsing and shampooing the bleach off. Because bleached hair produces unnatural looking warm tones such as red, orange, gold, and yellow, it is necessary to apply a tint (permanent color) afterwards to neutralize the red, orange and gold tones (See "Correcting Undesirable Hair Colors" on page 76) and a toner to neutralize the yellow and pale yellow tones. (See: "The Two-Step Method For Coloring Hair Light Blonde" on page 66). **The level at which you stop the lightening action will serve as your guideline in choosing the color level of your tint.**

Selecting And Applying Hair Color

You can follow this guide:

Black Hair Bleached to These Levels	Tint		Toner	
	Cool Tones	Warm Tones	Cool Tones	Warm Tones
2. Dark Red Brown	Dark Brown	Dark Auburn	—	—
3. Med. Red Brown	Med. Ash Brown	Med. Auburn	—	—
4. Red	Light Ash brown	Light Warm Brown	—	—
5. Orange	Dark Ash Blonde	Chestnut	—	—
6. Gold	Medium Blonde	Strawberry Blonde	Light Beige Blonde	Wheat Blonde
7. Yellow	—	—		Very Light Gold Blonde
8. Pale Yellow	—	—	Platinum Blonde	

How To Apply A Bleach

Step 1: Go over the list of "Setting Up to Color Your Hair at Home" on page 9.

Step 2: Buy two hair bleaching kits such as Ultra Blue Lady Clairol. Also buy the hair color you will need after bleaching. Don't shampoo your hair for at least 2 days before bleaching.

Step 3: Brush your dry hair through, making sure not to irritate the scalp. Apply vaseline around the hairline and ears. Put on a white towel, plastic cape and rubber gloves.

Step 4: Divide your hair into four sections by making a part from the middle of your forehead all the way over the crown down to the middle of your nape. Brush the hair to each side. Now make a part from the middle of your ear up to the top of the crown. Gather the hair from the quarter front section, twist it around and hold it together using a jaw. (A jaw is a clip which is extremely practical and often used by hair stylists). Do the same for the quarter section behind your ear. Make a part on the other side from the middle of your ear to the crown and pin up each section.

Selecting And Applying Hair Color

Dividing the hair into four sections will make it easier for you to properly apply the bleach. Use this method of applying bleach if your hair needs to be bleached from the roots to the ends. You may want to practice this method once by applying a creme rinse instead of bleach. You may also want to ask a friend to help you but make sure he/she reads the instructions first.

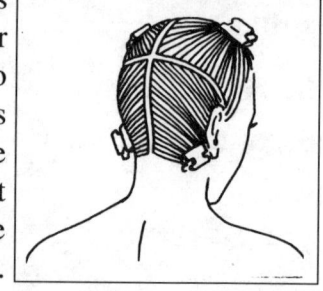

Step 5: Take one of the bleaching kits and empty the bleach, developer and activating powder into a glass bowl (size of a soup bowl), mixing well with a tint brush. Next, remove one of the clips pinning up a quarter section in the back of your head. Make a horizontal part with the pointy end of the tint brush about half an inch from the nape. Lift the upper part of the hair, twist it and hold it together with the clip. Using the tint brush, apply the bleach on three quarters of the length of the sectioned hair, leaving the first half inch from the scalp unbleached. The part of the hair closest to the scalp always bleaches faster than the rest because it is the newest, most virgin part of the hair. It is also the part most affected by the heat of the scalp which speeds up the lightening process. Make sure you saturate each section well and evenly with the bleach. Now remove the clip from the hair next to the section you just did. Again using the pointy end of the tint brush, make a horizontal part a half inch from the nape, just like the one you did next to it. Take the top part and clip it. Apply the bleach on about three quarters of the length of that section, not putting any bleach on the first half inch from the scalp. Work your way up to the crown, parting the hair horizontally in half inch wide

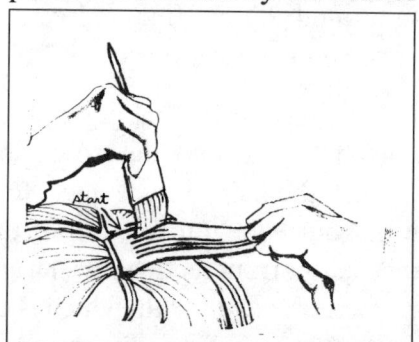

Selecting And Applying Hair Color

sections. Next come the front sides. Start at the temple in the same way you did the back of your head, parting the hair horizontally in half inch wide sections and putting the bleach on about three quarters of the length of the hair. The process of applying bleach should not take more than 15 minutes. Wait until the hair turns to an orange tone before mixing the bleach from the second bleaching kit.

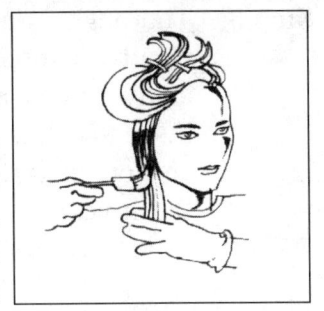

Step 6: Now apply the bleach on the roots. Since the roots lighten faster, you have given the ends a head start. By the time the roots turn a pale yellow, the ends will also be a pale yellow. As you section the hair to apply bleach on the roots, you may discover areas that are darker than orange. Re-apply bleach to these spots when you apply the bleach on the roots. It is important to get an even tone in order to get an even color with the toner (or tint) later. Using the pointy end of the tint brush, start applying the bleach by parting the hair from the middle of your forehead to the crown. Using the tint brush, cover the roots well and evenly. The next part is a half inch below. Part the hair again by sliding the pointy end of the brush horizontally along the scalp, the same length as the first part. You won't need to pin up the hair because the bleach in the ends will make the hair lie flat. Do one side at a time. When you have finished both sides, start at the crown on the back of your head, making a horizontal part again with the pointy end of the tint brush. Separate the hair and apply the bleach on the unbleached part. A half inch below make another section and so on until you reach the nape.

Step 7: When the bleach has lightened your hair to a yellow or pale yellow shade, it is time to rinse the bleach out of your hair. Should you find after shampooing that there are parts that are too dark, you will need to re-apply bleach to these spots and wait until they are as light as the rest.

Selecting And Applying Hair Color

Step 8: Thoroughly rinse the bleach out of your hair with warm water. Gently shampoo your hair once. Avoid rubbing your scalp and apply a creme rinse. Squeeze any excess water out of your hair into a towel. Dry your hair until it is just a bit damp. Wait about an hour before applying a toner so your scalp will be less sensitive. Bleaching your hair will cost about $12.00.

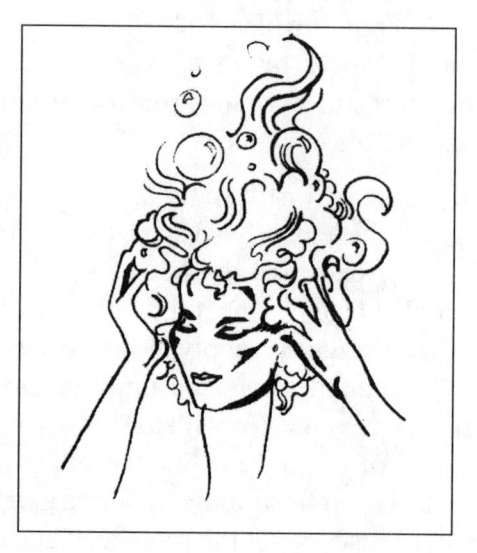

Brand Names: L'Oréal Super Blue Creme Oil Lightener
Super Blondissima Hair Lightener by l'Oréal

Selecting And Applying Hair Color

Testing For Allergic Reactions
Permanent Hair Color (Tint)

Although only 0.04% of the population is allergic to hair color, you can make absolutely sure that you are not one of these few by using the patch test 24 hours before coloring your hair. Unlike allergic reactions to food which can have very serious consequences, an allergic reaction to hair color is not life threatening. An allergic reaction to a tint can manifest itself in symptoms such as swelling of the face, headache, vomiting, itchy red spots or small blisters. If you exhibit any of these symptoms, you should see your doctor immediately. Given that prevention is always easier than a cure, it makes good sense to conduct a patch test before coloring your hair.

Step 1: Buy the hair coloring kit.

Step 2: Wash a small area, about the size of a dime, on the inside of your arm. Mix a capful of color with a capful of developer into a glass bowl. Stir the mixture with a Q-tip. Using the Q-tip, apply the color on the washed area of your arm. Leave the area uncovered for as long as possible. Then cover it, by loosely placing a band-aid over it and leave it for 24 hours. Wash off the color with soap and water. If you are allergic, the test area will be red, itchy and burn. Having an allergic reaction to a product does not mean that you will always have an allergic reaction to that product. Test yourself again at a later time.

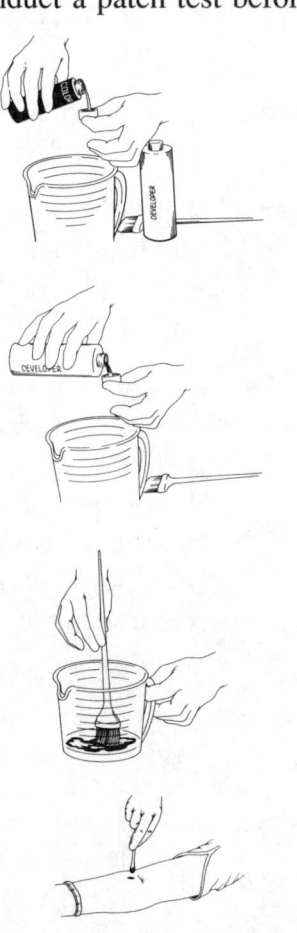

Selecting And Applying Hair Color

How To Test Your New Hair Color

Test your new hair color on a strand of hair before you apply the color all over your hair. There are two ways that you can test a strand. The first way involves cutting a strand of hair as close as possible to the roots. Put scotch tape around it, dip it into the color, let it process and rinse off the color. The problem with this method is that although it is held together with scotch tape, the strand easily comes apart. A further problem is that if you need to test another strand, you will need to cut another piece of hair. A more practical method involves pulling the strand of hair to be tested through a hole in the streaking cap.

Step 1: Go over the list of "Setting Up To Color Your Hair at Home" on page 9.

Step 2: Buy the coloring kit and any other accessories you will need to color your hair.

Step 3: Put the streaking cap over your dry hair. Using a crochet needle, pull out a strand, or two consisting of about 10 hairs, on top of your head.

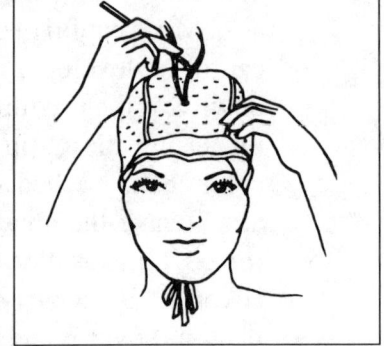

Step 4: Remove the bottle of hair color from the hair coloring kit. Fill the bottle cap with color and pour it into a glass bowl. Next fill the cap with developer and add it to the color. Using a tint brush, mix the color with the developer. Put the cap back on the bottle of hair color.

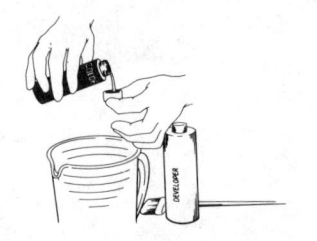

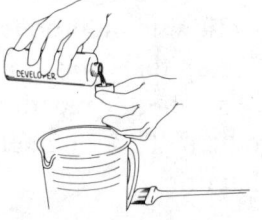

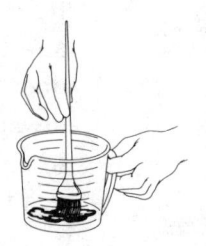

Selecting And Applying Hair Color

Using the tint brush, apply the color on the strand. Allow it to process for 30 minutes. (Even if the directions in the coloring kit recommend a processing time from 5 to 30 minutes, it is better to let it process for the full 30 minutes. The exception to this rule is bleach. For instance, if you bought a dark brown shade, the color will gradually reach that level. However, if you rinse it off after 5 or 10 minutes, you will not get a dark brown, but a shade much lighter).

Step 5: Without removing the cap, rinse the color off the strand and dry it with a hair blower. You can only properly judge hair color when hair is dry. Now you can see if you like the new color. If you are not satisfied with the color, you can buy another shade. You may also want to mix two shades together. (See "Customizing Your Hair Color" on page 72). In this case you will need to test another strand.

Techniques
The Professionals Use

Tinting White/Grey Hair Red

If your hair is more than 50% white, you will need to mix a basic shade (i.e. medium blonde, light brown, etc.) (See Color Chart on pg. 16.) with a red tone. Using a red color on its own such as mahogany, auburn, strawberry blonde, etc. would turn your white hair bright red. Make sure that both colors are on the same color level and not more than one level lighter or one level darker. For example, if you are combining mahogany and dark blonde, dark blonde would serve as the basic color and mahogany as the red tone. You would mix 3/4 bottle of mahogany, 1/4 bottle of dark blonde and 1 bottle of developer. ("Bottles" are generally 2 ounces)

What You Do When the Red Has Faded From the Ends

Of all the color tones, tinted red tones fade the fastest. As a result, when you tint the re-growth, you may also need to color the ends in order to intensify the red tone. A good way to do this is to mix two formulas. One formula is for the roots, containing both the red tone and the base color. The second formula only has the red tone. Both of these formulas should be mixed at the same time.

Formula for the re-growth: Mix 3/4 bottle of mahogany with 1/4 bottle of dark blonde with an equal amount of developer (1 bottle).

Formula for the ends: Mix 1/2 bottle of mahogany with 1/2 bottle of developer.

- Apply the formula on the re-growth.
- After 15 minutes, apply the formula on the ends, allowing it to process for another 15 minutes.

By allowing the second formula to stand before using it, you minimize the action of the peroxide (developer) leaving you only with the color molecules which are deposited into your hair. With the exception of the re-growth, the rest of the hair has color that just needs to be intensified.

Techniques The Professionals Use

How To Highlight Your Hair

If you want to brighten your hair color, either by giving it a natural look or by creating a dramatic look, but only want to color it a few times a year, then highlighting is for you.

The easiest method for highlighting hair is to use a cap as well as a special bleach (streaking/frosting kit). Hair colorists have been using this technique for years because it is practical, safe, and can be used on both tinted and untinted hair. The tone and degree of lightness will be different for each color-type. This is an important point to consider if you want your highlights to suit you. (See: "Know Your Color-Type" on page 16).

Step 1: Get everything ready for coloring your hair such as a plastic cape, glass bowl, tint brush, etc. (See: Setting Up to Color Your Hair at Home on page 9).

Step 2: Buy two streaking kits to ensure that you do not run out of color.

Step 3: **You are now ready to test a strand.** Brush your dry, unwashed hair back. Put a streaking cap over your head. Using the crochet needle, pull out a couple of strands on top of your head, each strand containing about 20 hairs.

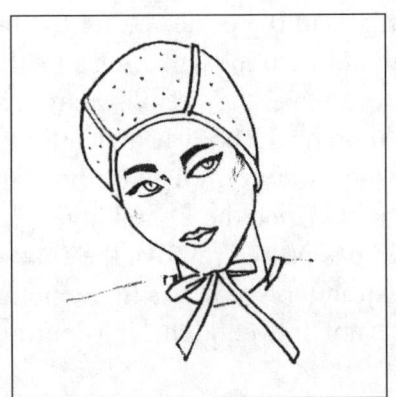

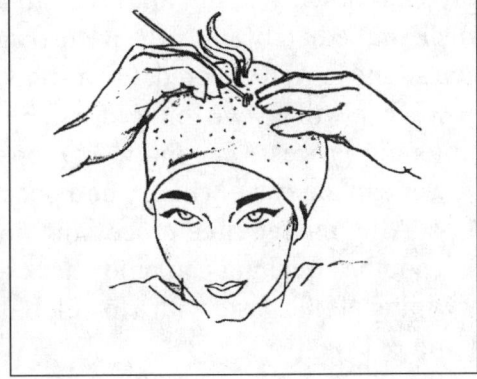

Techniques The Professionals Use

Step 4: In a glass bowl mix a small amount of bleaching powder with a small amount of developing lotion. The consistency should resemble that of a creamy paste. Using a tint brush, apply the mixture on the strands, saturating them well.

Step 5: As you will see later, depending on your color-type, the color can be left on your hair from 5 to 60 minutes. If you hair is very dark, you may need to re-apply the bleach in order to make it light enough. After the desired amount of time, wipe off the bleach and dry the strands as well as you can with a towel. See if you like the color. You may need to re-apply the bleach (mix a fresh batch) to get a lighter color.

When you have achieved the lightness you want, rinse the color off the strands, remove the cap and blow dry the strands. You can better judge the effect when you see how the strands blend in with the rest of your hair. Depending on how you like the color, you may decide to change the timing when you highlight the rest of your head.

After you have completed the strand test, you can pull out the desired strands. Mix the powder bleach and the developer in a glass or porcelain bowl. Use the tint brush to mix it into a paste. Using the tint brush, immediately apply the paste on all of the strands, making sure that each strand is well covered. Put a shower cap over the streaking cap. The shower cap will do two things. First, by trapping the body heat it helps the lightening process. Secondly, it keeps the mixture moist. Without the shower cap the paste will dry and once it has dried the lightening action stops. After the required processing time has passed remove the shower cap (not the streaking cap) and check a strand to see if it is light enough by wiping off the paste with a towel. If it is not light enough, let it continue to process.

When it comes time to rinse off the paste take off the shower cap, but leave on the streaking cap. Rinse with warm water and apply a creme rinse on the strands which makes it easier to remove the streaking cap. Remove the streaking cap, rinse and shampoo. Apply a protein conditioner.

Techniques The Professionals Use

How long should you let the color process?

This depends on your color-type. Just remember the following rule of thumb: if you are a cool color-type, your highlights should also be cool, (in other words they should be a pale yellow) and if you are a warm color-type, your highlights should be warm (in other words red, gold or yellow). (See: "Know Your Color-Type" on page 16).

a) **The strong cool color-type** (winter) should highlight only a few strands around the face in order to create a dramatic effect. Of the four color-types, this color-type is least suited for highlights. Having a hair color that is naturally dark makes it harder to lighten strands to a pale yellow. Processing time may take up to one hour.

> **NOTE:**
> The pale yellow strands look more natural if you apply a toner after the lightening process is completed.

Here is what you do: When you buy your streaking kit, you should also buy a toner. But don't buy a toner that is silver or platinum blonde, because it will make your highlights look like grey hair. What you want is a toner that will make your lightened hair beige blonde. The right shade for instance, should be a pearl ash blonde which is made by L'Oreal and called "Excellence". You apply the toner after washing off the bleach. (Remember to keep on your streaking cap). Mix the toner according to the instructions and apply it on the strands with a tint brush. Allow it to process for the required time. (Usually between 20 to 30 minutes) Then rinse, apply a creme rinse and pull off the cap. Rinse your hair, shampoo and apply a protein conditioner.

b) **The soft-cool color-type** (summer) looks wonderful with a lot of highlights. They should be lightened to a yellow or pale yellow color. Highlighting is actually the best way of coloring hair for this color-type. Don't be concerned about the "yellow". Once the highlights blend in with the rest of the hair, they will look like light beige blonde, rather than yellow. Processing time should be between 15 and 45 minutes.

> **NOTE:**
> If your hair is dark ash blonde see above note.

Techniques The Professionals Use

c) **If you are a strong-warm color-type** (autumn), your hair can be lightened to dark red, red, light red or copper.
Processing time should be between 5 and 15 minutes.

d) **The soft-warm color-type** (spring) can have highlights in light copper and gold tones. The processing time is between 5 and 15 minutes.

You can highlight your hair in two different ways. One way will give the impression that your hair color is lighter all over. To create this effect, you pull thin strands (about 10 hairs per strand) out of each hole in the streaking cap. (You should not do this if you are a strong-cool color-type).

The second method will make the highlights stand out more. Use thicker strands (about 20 hairs per strand but only one strand per square inch). Pull out fewer strands if you have less hair and more if you have a lot of hair.

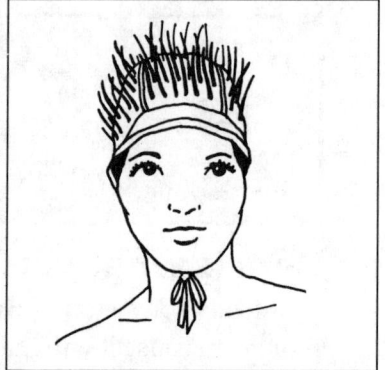

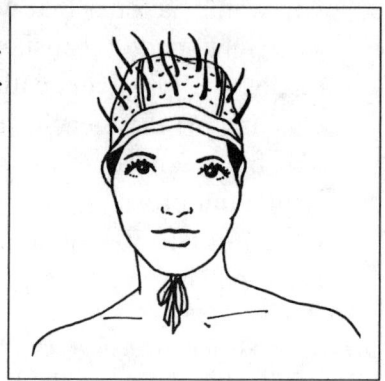

Techniques The Professionals Use

Brand Names of Highlighting Kits:
- L'Oréal Frosting Kit
- Frost & Tip Kit by Clairol
- Frost & Glow by Revlon
- Light Effects by Clairol

Light Effects also comes in a kit with a plastic cap, crochet needle, etc. The difference between this kit and a Frost & Glow kit is in the lightening solution. It is designed to produce subtle highlights which means that it will make your own hair color only a little lighter and has very little effect on tinted hair and can only be used on untinted hair.

Highlighting your hair yourself will cost between $10.00 and $15.00.

Techniques The Professionals Use

The Two-Step Method For Coloring Your Hair Light Blonde

Two-step hair coloring, also known as double-process blonding is the hair coloring technique necessary to achieve those very light pastel blonde hair colors associated with Marilyn Monroe and Jean Harlow. This two-step method is the only technique that makes it possible to change dark hair to platinum blonde or to very light beige blonde.

> **NOTE:**
> If your hair color is medium blonde or light blonde, you can use Miss Clairol "Extra Lightening Hair Color" or Excellence by L'Oréal in shades such as Ultra Light Ash Blonde or Ultra Light Beige Blonde. However, if you use these shades on darker hair, you will end up with a gold/brassy tone.

The first step involves bleaching hair to a pale yellow shade. (The yellow of a lemon). Only with pale yellow bleached hair as the base color is it possible to achieve a pastel blonde tone. The second step involves applying a toner which will change the pale yellow color to a pastel blonde tone. Pastel blonde tones are very light soft blonde shades. Toners are hair colors that are applied on very light bleached hair in order to create pastel blonde shades. No other type of hair color should be used. The entire coloring process will take approximately 2 hours and cost approximately $15.00.

Step 1: Bleach your hair to a pale yellow. (See: "Bleach" Pre-Lightening on page 52). Dry your hair until it feels damp.

Step 2: Buy a toner kit in the drugstore. There are two types of toners - one that is a permanent type color and the other that is a semi-permanent rinse. The advantage of using a permanent type color toner is the number of different shades available from different manufacturers. Although the semi-permanent rinse toner has fewer shades to choose from, it tends to be gentler on your hair. A popular brand is Born Blonde by Clairol.

Techniques The Professionals Use

Step 3: Apply the toner on your damp, pale yellow bleached hair. Using the applicator bottle, saturate your entire head with the toner, gently working the color into your hair without rubbing it into your scalp.

If the toner looks dark on your hair, don't be afraid. It is normal. Just remember that if your toner kit is a very light ash blonde or platinum blonde, the color will never become

> **NOTE:**
> If you find that the color burns your scalp, add 1/2 ounce of club soda to the toner formula.

darker than that particular shade. As a rule, it is better to err on the side of leaving the color on for a longer period of time. "Born Blonde's" toner recommends leaving the toner on between 15 and 45 minutes. Remember that the toner's job is to deposit color into your hair, and if it is not given enough time to process, your hair color will remain too yellow.

Step 4: Rinse, shampoo and apply a protein conditioner.

The next time you bleach your hair, apply the bleach only on the roots. Be careful not to get the bleach on the already bleached part of your hair. Bleach is very hard on your hair and repeated bleaching of the same area will cause the hair to break off.

Using a tint brush, apply the toner on the roots. (See: "How to Apply a Tint" on page 43). You can overlap the toner and if your hair color has faded or has become somewhat yellow, you can put the toner on the rest of the hair for the last 10 minutes of the processing time.

Brands of Hair Toners:
- Pastel Blonde by L'Oréal
- Creme Toner by Clairol
- Born Blonde Lotion Toner by Clairol
- Naturally Blonde by Clairol

Techniques The Professionals Use

Lowlighting

Lowlighting, as the word suggests, is the opposite of highlighting. Instead of making hair lighter, it makes strands of hair darker. This technique can be applied on white hair to give it more color. It is a natural and economical way of adding color to white hair without having to color the roots every four to six weeks.

Step 1: Get ready to color your hair at home by going over the section on "Setting Up to Color Your Hair at Home" on page 9.

Step 2: Buy Clairesse by Clairol hair coloring kit. This particular hair color contains no ammonia, making the color last longer without becoming lighter or brassy. It is a cross between a permanent and semi-permanent color. (See "Semi-Permament Hair Color-Category II" on page 35). Lowlighting is done only a few times a year whereas tinted hair is re-touched every four to eight weeks. However, when the lowlights fade, the same strands cannot be re-colored because it is impossible to select the same strands twice. It is therefore important to choose a type of hair color that does not fade quickly. Shades such as dark and medium brown are best suited for lowlighting white hair. (Of course if your pigmented hair is lighter, you should not use these dark shades).

Step 3: Brush your dry, unwashed hair back and put the streaking cap on your head. Mix a little bit of color to test a strand. Leave it on for 30 minutes (See: "How to Test Your New Hair Color" on page 58). After you have completed the strand test, pull out strands with the crochet needle at the rate of 10 hairs at a time (3 strands per square inch). Pour the color and the developer into a glass bowl and mix it with a tint brush. Now use the tint brush to apply the color on the strands, saturating them well. Wait 30 minutes, rinse the color off, apply some conditioner and gently remove the plastic cap. Rinse, shampoo and apply a creme rinse.

Techniques The Professionals Use

A second use of the lowlighting technique is to put dark strands of color in hair that has too many highlights. The lowlighting technique can be used to give hair more contrast. Lowlighting can also be used to gradually return bleached blonde hair to its natural color. Instead of coloring all the hair dark right away, adding dark strands will make your hair color darker and softer. (See: "Coloring Your Bleached Hair Back to its Natural Color" on page 70).

Techniques The Professionals Use

Coloring Your Light Blonde Bleached Or Tinted Hair Back To Its Natural Color

Wait until you have a regrowth and use your natural shade as your guide for buying hair color. (See: "How You Can Determine What Level Your Hair Color Is" on page 15).

Step 1: Get ready to color your hair. Read the section on "Setting Up to Color Your Hair at Home" on page 9. Buy two permanent hair coloring kits such as "Excellence" by L'Oréal and any other accessories you need. Avoid choosing an ash tone.

Step 2: Test a strand. Put the streaking cap over your dry, unwashed hair. Pull out a strand on top of your head. Pour one cap full of hair color (no developer) into a glass measuring cup. Using the tint brush, apply it on the strand, saturating it well with color. Leave it on for 15 minutes. The purpose of using the color alone without the developer is to put a "filler" into the hair first. Very light bleached hair needs pigments and base colors such as light brown, dark blonde, etc. contain all of the basic pigments. Putting a "filler" into the hair first helps prevent the new hair color from fading later on.

Now, using the tint brush, mix one cap full of hair color with one cap full of developer. Apply it over the "filler" on the strand of hair. Wait 30 minutes before rinsing the color off the strand. Dry it using a blow dryer. Remove the cap and see if you like the color. You may want to apply a darker or lighter shade for which you will of course have to make another trip to the drugstore.

Step 3: Brush your dry hair back and put the streaking cap over your head. Using the crochet needle, pull the strands through all the holes in the cap. Pour the entire bottle of hair color into the glass measuring cup. Using the tint brush, apply this "filler" on all of the strands. Leave it on for 15 minutes.

Techniques The Professionals Use

Step 4: Take the bottle of hair color from the second coloring kit and pour it into the glass bowl adding the bottle of developer. Use the tint brush to stir the mixture. Apply this formula over the "filler" leaving it on for 30 minutes.

Step 5: Rinse the color off the strands, apply shampoo and take off the streaking cap. Rinse your hair and shampoo lightly. Apply a protein conditioner.

> **NOTE:**
> If you want to color all of your light blonde hair back to its natural color, you should not use the streaking cap. In this case, apply the filler all over your hair using an applicator bottle, and working the color into your hair evenly. After 15 minutes, mix the hair color and the developer in the applicator bottle and apply the formula over the filler. Leave it on your hair for 30 minutes.

Techniques The Professionals Use

Customizing Your Hair Color

This technique is used only with permanent hair color (tints). (See: "Permanent Hair Color" on page 41).

Although one shade of hair color is usually enough, you can sometimes get a better result by mixing two shades. (It is not necessary to use more than two colors). Professional hair colorists use this technique. In the long run, using two colors and therefore two coloring kits is no more expensive than using one kit. You simply keep the unmixed color for the next time you color your hair. After mixing a certain amount of each hair color and developer into a separate applicator bottle or glass measuring cup, (See: "Setting Up to Color Your Hair at Home" on page 9) put the cap back on the unused portion of the bottle, closing it tightly. The tint that has been mixed with the developer cannot be re-used after one hour.

When is it appropriate to mix two different shades?

1. When your hair is more than 25% white and you color your hair in a red, gold or ash tone.

2. When you want your new color not to be too dark or too ash, red or gold.

Important points to remember when customizing your hair color formula

1. Use only one brand of hair color. Do not mix different brands, or different products from the same company.

2. Use two shades that are similar - shades that are one level lighter or darker or on the same level (medium brown with medium auburn, or light blonde with light golden blonde). (See: Chart of Hair Color Levels and Tones on page 16).

Techniques The Professionals Use

3. Use a color chart as your guide.
4. Avoid mixing ash tones with gold or red tones (See: "A Little Bit of Color Theory" on page 74).
5. Mix a neutral or base color such as medium blonde or dark brown with a warm tone such as red or gold or with a cool tone such as ash or silver.

Examples Of Mixing Two Different Hair Colors

Buy two hair coloring kits; use the equivalent of 1 bottle of hair color (2 oz.) and 1 bottle of developer (2 oz.)

Your Own Hair Color is:	Warm Tone Mix:	Cool Tone Mix:
More than 25% white and the rest is dark brown	1/2 bottle dark brown 1/2 bottle dark auburn 1 bottle developer	1/2 bottle dark brown 1/2 bottle med. brown 1 bottle developer
More than 25% white and the rest is light brown	3/4 bottle light auburn 1/4 bottle light brown 1 bottle developer	1/2 bottle light ash brown 1/2 bottle light brown 1 bottle developer
More then 25% white and the rest is dark ash blonde		1/2 bottle dark blonde 1/2 bottle med. ash blonde 1 bottle developer
More than 25% white and the rest is med. ash blonde		3/4 bottle light ash blonde 1/4 bottle med. blonde 1 bottle developer
100% white - before it turned white it was a strawberry blonde	3/4 bottle reddish blonde 1/4 bottle med. blonde 1 bottle developer	
Bleached pale yellow		3/4 bottle platinum blonde 1/4 bottle light beige blonde

IMPORTANT
Always write down the formula you use so that you can duplicate it or make changes if necessary.

Techniques The Professionals Use

Know A Little Bit Of Color Theory
The Color Wheel

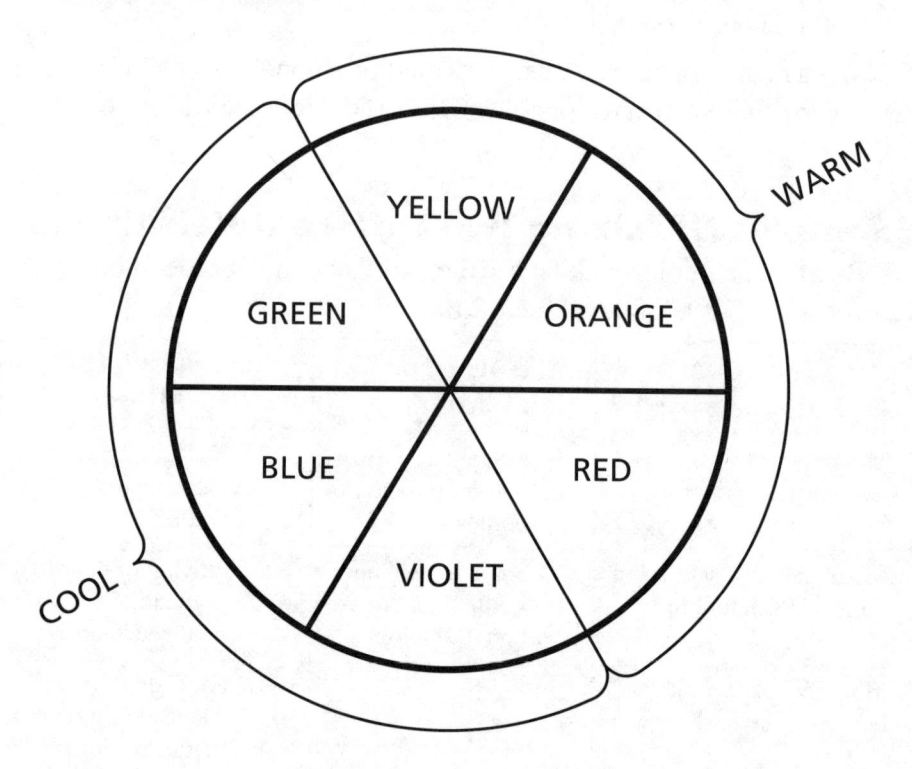

(Color wheel diagram showing YELLOW, GREEN, ORANGE, BLUE, RED, VIOLET segments; WARM side on the right, COOL side on the left)

Just as your own hair color is made up of different colored pigments, permanent hair color consists of different colored pigments. Since permanent hair color is the most versatile of all the types of hair color, some knowledge of color theory is helpful. Permanent hair color comes in basic shades such as light blonde, medium brown, etc. in warm tones such as gold blonde, mahogany, copper, etc. and in cool tones such as ash blonde, etc. If the majority of pigments in a hair color - be it natural or artificial - are red or gold, the hair color is considered a warm color, as seen in tones such as copper, mahogany, chestnut, auburn, gold blonde,etc. The majority of these pigments are either yellow, orange or red. An ash hair color, such as light ash blonde, smoky blonde, etc. is considered a cool tone and contains many green or blue pigments, whereas a silver

Techniques The Professionals Use

blonde hair color contains many violet pigments. Permanent hair colors that have an equal amount of warm and cool pigments are considered neutral (basic shades such as light brown, medium blonde, black, etc.) See "Chart of Hair Color Levels and Tones" on page 16. Now have a look at the color wheel. **Each of the warm colors has a cool color opposite it and vice versa.** If you were to take an equal amount of red and mix it with an equal amount of green, the result would be a neutral color, neither red nor green, but brown. The same applies to orange which has blue as its opposite color and yellow which has violet as its opposite color. Knowing this basic law of color will help you choose the right color, correct unwanted hair colors and custom mix your hair color the right way.

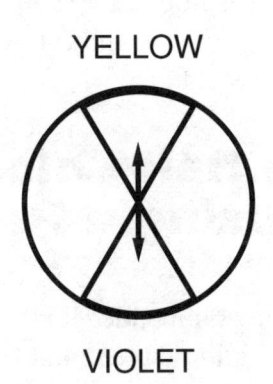

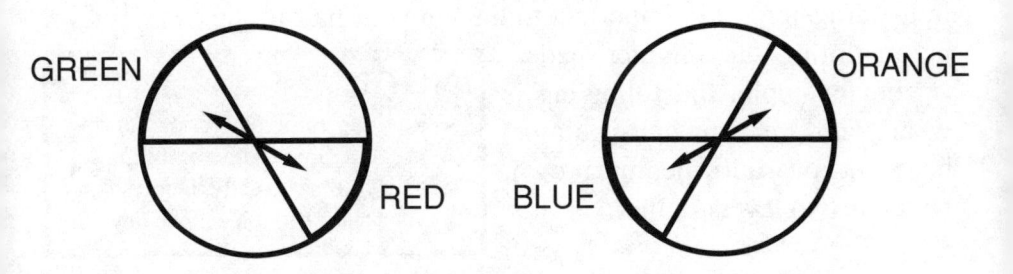

NOTE:
A tone describes colors such as ash (cool), red or gold (warm).

YELLOW

VIOLET

GREEN

ORANGE

RED   BLUE

75

Correcting Undesirable Hair Colors

How To Correct Undesirable Hair Colors

What can you do when you have used the wrong color on your hair. Imagine that your hair is too dark, or looks green, or the Henna you used is too red, or your blonde hair has become too yellow. Well, you can make your own color corrections.

Correcting a Hair Color that is too Dark or too Red After Using a Semi-Permanent Rinse.

(Category I, see: "Semi-Permanent Rinse" on page 30).

Should the color not wash out after several shampoos, you can buy Metalex by Clairol at the drugstore and follow the product instructions. The cost is approximately $5.00.

Correcting a Hair Color that is too Dark After Using a Permanent Hair Color.

This technique is also recommended for the long-lasting semi-permanent hair color. Since it is impossible to lighten tinted hair with another tint, you will need to use a soft bleach to lighten your hair before applying a permanent hair color in a lighter shade. Always refer to the color chart in the drugstore. It is important to lighten your hair to the desired level before tinting it to a lighter shade.

For example, the following is what you do if your hair is almost black but you want a medium brown, which is two levels lighter.

> **NOTE:**
> Make your color corrections during the day. Daylight is the best light for judging colors correctly. Don't shampoo your hair for at least one day.

Correcting Undesirable Hair Colors

Step 1: Buy two hair lightener kits (one may not be enough) such as Super Blondissima by L'Oréal. (See: "The Different Stages Of Bleaching Hair And The Corresponding Tint Shades" on 78). Also buy two permanent hair color kits such as Excellence by L'Oréal, in medium ash brown. Make sure that you have all the other accessories for coloring your hair at home. Go over the section on "Setting up to Color Your Hair at Home" to prepare for coloring your hair.

Step 2: First test a strand. Brush your dry, unwashed hair back with a few strokes only. Put a plastic streaking cap firmly over your head. Now using the crochet needle, pull out a strand of hair consisting of about 20 hairs through one of the holes in the cap. Pull out another strand next to it. This gives you more hair to work with and makes it easier to judge the color later. The strands should be where you can see them well like close to the front of your face or on top of your head.

Take the two bottles out of the hair lightener kit. Fill one cap with lightener liquid and another cap with developer. Using a tint brush, mix the two solutions in a glass bowl. Apply the mixture on three quarters of your hair, leaving an inch from the scalp untouched for now. The reason for doing this is that the hair closest to the scalp is the most recently grown hair and lightens faster than the rest. Cover the bowl. Check the color after 5 minutes by wiping off the bleach with a towel. If it is not light enough, apply more lightener. The color of the strand should be a dark red brown. Check the color in another 5 minutes. When the color has turned dark red brown, you are ready to apply the bleach on the roots. Leave it on for 10 minutes and check. When your hair has turned medium red brown, rinse, shampoo and towel dry the strands. (Don't remove the streaking cap yet). Dry the strands with a hair dryer.

When hair is made lighter, it goes through different color levels and tones. Black hair goes from dark red brown to medium red brown to light reddish brown to light red to orange to gold-yellow and finally to a pale yellow.

Correcting Undesirable Hair Colors

The Different Stages Of Bleaching Hair and The Corresponding Tint Shades.

Natural Hair Color	Desired Color	Desired Color	Desired Color	Desired Color	Desired Color	Desired Color
Black	Dark Brown	Medium Brown	Light Brown	Dark Blonde	Medium Blonde	Light Blonde
Bleach Hair to:	Dark Red Brown	Med. Red Brown	Light Red Brown	Orange	Gold	Yellow
Apply This Tint After Bleaching:	Dark Brown	Med. Ash Brown	Light Ash Brown	Dark Ash Blonde	Medium Ash Blonde	Light Beige Blonde
For a Warm Tone:	Dark Auburn	Medium Auburn	Light Auburn	Light Chestnut	Medium Gold Blonde	Light Blonde

NOTE:
Hair bleached to red or gold needs to have a permanent hair color applied. Pale yellow bleached hair needs a toner to give it pigments.

Step 3: Rinse the bowl containing the remaining bleach, as well as the tint brush. Mix one capful of medium ash brown and one capful of developer into the bowl and blend it together, using the tint brush. Using the tint brush, apply the tint on the strands. Process for 30 minutes. Leave the cap on, rinse, shampoo, towel dry and blow dry the strands. (To accurately judge hair color you need to have dry hair). See if you are satisfied with the color. The extra hour you spend doing a strand test is time well spent. You are now ready to do your whole head.

Correcting Undesirable Hair Colors

If you do not want a warm tone in your hair, then make sure to choose a shade with an ash tone. Ash as you know from reading "Know A Little Bit of Color Theory"

> **NOTE:**
> Always lighten your hair to the level necessary for the lighter color you want. Check the color chart in the drugstore and find out what a dark brown, medium brown, etc. actually looks like. Once you are sure of what you want, go ahead with it.

on page 74 contains green which neutralizes red.

Step 4: Now lighten all your hair. Using a glass bowl mix the bleach according to the product instructions. However, only use half of the amounts indicated. Keep the other half for later.

Lightly dampen your hair with a spray bottle. Divide your hair into four sections by making a part from the middle of your forehead all the way over the crown and down to the middle of your nape. Brush the hair to each side. Now make a part from the middle of your ear up to the top of the crown. Gather the hair from the quarter front section, twist it around and hold it up with a large clip. (Hairdressers use "jaws" for this purpose.) Do the same for the quarter section behind your ear. Make a part on the other side from the middle of your ear to the crown and pin each section up. Dividing the hair into four sections will make it easier for you to properly apply the bleach.

Remove one of the clips holding together a quarter section in the back of your head. Using the pointy end of the tint brush, make a horizontal part about half an inch from the nape. Lift the upper part of the hair, twist it around and clip it again.

Using the tint brush, apply the bleach on three quarters of the length of the sectioned hair, leaving the first half inch from the scalp without bleach. The part of the hair closest to the scalp always bleaches faster than the rest. This is because it is the newest, most virgin part of your hair. It is also most affected by the warmth of the scalp which speeds up the lightening process.

Correcting Undesirable Hair Colors

Make sure you saturate each section well and evenly so you don't have areas of different color. Now remove the clip from the hair next to the section you just did. Again using the pointy end of the tint brush make a part a half inch from the nape, just like the one next to it. Take the top part and clip it up again. Apply the bleach on about three quarters of the length of that section, not putting any bleach on the first half inch form the scalp. Work your way up to the crown, horizontally parting hair in half inch wide sections.

Next come the front and sides. Start at the temple in the same manner you did the back of your head, parting the hair horizontally in half inch wide sections and putting the bleach on about three quarters of the length of the hair. If you need more bleach mix the remaining bleach in your hair lightener kit (you still have one kit left). The application should not take more than 10 to 15 minutes. You may want a friend to help you.

Given your experience with the strand test, you should know how long it takes your color to turn dark red brown. Although you may ultimately want to lighten your hair to a medium red brown color (the base color to put on a medium ash brown tint) the ends need only be a dark red brown for now. Since the roots lighten faster, you have already given the ends a 10 minute headstart. By the time the roots turn a medium red brown, the ends will also be a medium red brown.

NOTE: Should you have bleached your hair lighter than medium red brown, you can still put on a medium ash brown tint and the color will still turn out fine.

Step 5: When the color has turned a dark red brown, you should apply the bleach on the roots. Mix the bleach from the second bleaching kit. This time start applying the bleach by parting the hair on top of your head. Using the pointy end of the tint brush, part your hair from the middle of your forehead to the crown. Using the tint brush cover the roots well and evenly. The next part is a half

Correcting Undesirable Hair Colors

inch below. Part the hair again by sliding the pointy end of the brush horizontally along the scalp, the same length as the first part. You won't need to pin up the hair because the bleach that is already on the ends will make the hair lie flat. Do one side at a time.

When you have finished both sides, start at the crown and do the back of your head by making a horizontal part. Apply the bleach on the roots. Half an inch below make another horizontal part, and continue sectioning the hair until you reach the nape. This application should not take longer than 10 minutes.

When the roots have reached the same color level as the ends, thoroughly rinse off the bleach, shampoo once without rubbing the scalp and apply a creme rinse. Towel dry and comb your hair through with a wide-tooth comb.

Step 6: Mix the medium ash brown color into the applicator bottle. Shake the bottle holding it away from your eyes and snip the tip off. (You may want to mix the color into your own applicator bottle). Apply the color with the applicator bottle. If you have very short hair, you can squeeze the color on your head, gently working it into the hair with your other hand, and making sure that all the hair is saturated with color.

If your hair is longer, make parts half an inch apart with the nozzle of the applicator bottle, starting on top of your head. To make sure that every part has color you will need to do this systematically. You can also use the tint brush, using the technique for applying bleach to the root area. Bring the color all the way through the hair, from the scalp to the ends. Using a wide-tooth comb, gently comb the color through your hair, starting from the nape and moving up to the top of your head. Allow the color to process for 30 minutes. Rinse well, shampoo once and apply a protein conditioner.

NOTE:
Don't forget to put Vaseline on the skin around your hairline before you color your hair.

Correcting Undesirable Hair Colors

Correcting Dark Ends On Tinted Hair

Dark ends are usually the result of applying a tint all over your hair from roots to ends every time you color your hair. This method which puts a tint on top of a tint makes the ends very porous and makes the color darker and darker with every application. As previously mentioned, an artficial pigment cannot lighten another artificial pigment. You cannot use a tint of a lighter shade to lighten dark ends. You will first have to lighten the ends with a soft bleach and then color your hair with the shade you use on the rest of your hair. In the future only color the regrowth. (See: "How to Apply A Tint" on page 43).

Step 1: Postpone the color correction until you have a regrowth and you need to tint your hair. Buy a hair lightener kit in a shade you usually use. Make sure you have the necessary accessories handy. Read the section on "Setting up to Color Your Hair at Home" on page 9.

Step 2: Mix the hair lightener. Test a strand as outlined in "Correcting a Hair Color that is too Dark After Using a Permanent Hair Color" on page 76. Apply the lightener on the part of the hair that is too dark. Lift the color one or two levels. If the ends of your hair are now dark brown and the rest of your hair is light brown, then lighten the ends to a light red brown. Refer to the chart on page 78 "The Different Stages of Levels of Bleaching Hair".

Step 3: After the strand has been lightened one or two levels, apply the tint. Again refer to the strand test previously mentioned.

Step 4: Apply the lightener on all of the ends using the application technique outlined in "Correcting a Hair Color that is Too Dark After Using a Permanent Hair Color" on page 76). Given your experience with the strand test, you should know how long it will take for your color to turn a couple of levels lighter.

Correcting Undesirable Hair Colors

Step 5: Rinse off the lightener, shampoo and apply a creme rinse. Gently towel dry your hair. Take the tint from the hair coloring kit and mix it into an applicator bottle. Put vaseline around your hairline. Using the applicator bottle, squeeze the color on your hair, making sure every hair from the roots to the ends is saturated with color. Allow the color to process for 30 minutes. Rinse, shampoo and apply a protein conditioner.

The cost of this color correction is approximately $20.00.

Correcting Undesirable Hair Colors

Correcting A Brassy/Reddish Hair Color

Tinted hair (permanent hair color) frequently becomes brassy. To neutralize the brassiness, you need to use a shade with an ash tone such as light ash brown, dark ash blonde, etc.

Step 1: Buy two hair coloring kits in an ash tone (in case one is not enough). L'Oréal (Excellence and Haute Mode) has a good choice of ash shades. Refer to the color selection chart in the drugstore.

Step 2: Using the applicator bottle, apply the tint over your entire head. Make sure every hair is covered with color. Process for 30 minutes. The next time you need to tint the re-growth, make sure you choose a shade with an ash tone and apply the color only on the re-growth. (See: "How to Apply a Tint" on page 43). The cost of this color correction is approximately $10.00.

Correcting Undesirable Hair Colors

Correcting A Hair Color That Is Too Gold/Brassy

When hair such as dark, medium and light brown has been tinted with a shade several levels lighter, the color is usually gold and brassy. Hair coloring technology is still not sufficiently advanced for us to be able to change dark hair to a beautiful light blonde shade without gold, brassiness in one step. To remedy this unnatural looking hair color, you need to change your tint formula to a darker shade.

> **NOTE:**
> The only time you can use a high-lifting tint is when your own hair color is not darker than dark blonde.

For example, if your natural hair color is dark brown, the color you choose should not be any lighter than dark ash blonde. Always use a shade with an ash tone. The ash will help to prevent brassiness.

Step 1: Buy a tinting kit that is at least two levels darker than the shade you used before. For example, if your natural hair color is medium or light brown and you used very light blonde, you will need to use medium ash blonde.

Step 2: Get ready to color your hair. Put on a plastic cape, apply vaseline around your hairline, etc. Don't shampoo your hair for at least one day. Mix the hair color (medium ash blonde for example) into the applicator bottle. Apply the color on your dry hair gently working the tint through your entire hair. (Avoid rubbing it into the scalp). Using a wide-tooth comb, gently comb your hair through starting at the nape. Allow the color to process for 30 minutes. Rinse, shampoo and apply a protein conditioner.

> **NOTE:**
> If you want light blonde hair and your hair is darker than dark blonde, you will need to use the two-step method. (See "The Two-Step Method for Coloring Your Hair Light Blonde" on page 66).

Step 3: When you need to color your re-growth, use the same shade for applying the tint on the roots. (See: "How to Apply a Tint" on page 43).

Correcting Undesirable Hair Colors

Correcting A Hair Color That Is Too Yellow

Hair that has been bleached but did not have a toner applied after bleaching (or was improperly colored) is the main cause of this unnatural looking hair color. Using a temporary rinse is not the way to change the yellow tone into a more natural looking hair color. A temporary rinse is too weak to neutralize the yellow to a beautiful blonde tone. Since the ends are usually lighter and more porous than the rest of the hair, a temporary rinse will only change the color of the ends to a silvery tone and give you a color that is uneven. The best way is to apply a toner such as a pastel blonde color for prelightened hair.

Step 1: Buy a toner kit. Choose a toner based on your color-type. If you are a soft-warm color-type, look for very light beige blonde or deep beige blonde. If you are a cool color-type, look for platinum blonde or light ash blonde.

Step 2: Apply the toner on your slightly damp hair, saturating the hair well with color.

Correcting Undesirable Hair Colors

Correcting Tinted Hair That Has Become "Green"

When an ash tone is applied to yellowish blonde hair as a way of neutralizing the yellow, the result is a greenish looking tone. Most people incorrectly put ash tones on yellow hair. If you refer to the color wheel in the section "A Little Bit of Color Theory" on page 74, you will notice that ash contains green pigments and neutralizes red, not yellow. The ash tone therefore is too strong for the yellowish base color and will show through with a greenish color. Since you want a nice blonde shade, you cannot put a red tone over the unwanted tone because it will make the color too dark. (As you can see on the color wheel, the opposite color of green is red - therefore neutralizing each other).

The solution for removing the green cast is to use a soft bleach (you can buy a Hair Lightener Kit in the drugstore) and apply a tint or toner afterwards depending on the color level you need.

Step 1: Test a strand. (See: "How to Test Your Hair Color" on page 57 Use the bleach and tint or toner as outlined below).

Step 2: Mix the bleach in an applicator bottle. Pour the creme or oil bleach, the developer and only 1/4 of the envelope containing the activator into the applicator bottle.

Step 3: Using the applicator bottle, apply the lightener all over your hair, starting at the nape. This should not take more than a couple of minutes. Leave the bleach on only for a few minutes, just long enough for the greenish cast to be eliminated.

Step 4: Rinse, shampoo once, apply a creme rinse and towel dry.

Step 5: Apply the hair color. If your hair is somewhere between medium blonde and light blonde, you can apply a tint in shades of medium blonde, light blonde and very light blonde. (No ash tones). If your hair is a bleached pale yellow, use a toner. (Toner kit). Apply the tint or toner all over your hair, using the applicator bottle. Allow the color to process for 30 minutes. Rinse, shampoo and apply a protein conditioner.

Correcting Undesirable Hair Colors

Correcting The Color Of Light Blonde Hair

Discoloration Due to Swimming

If the greenish cast does not come out after shampooing, use the following solution in your hair. Add one cup of lemon juice and one cup of Epsom salt to one gallon of distilled water. Mix well and let the mixture stand uncovered for 24 hours. Pour it over your hair, leaving it on for 30 minutes before rinsing with water.

Correcting Undesirable Hair Colors

How To Remove Henna From Your Hair

Although a Henna color only coats hair, it stays in your hair for a very long time requiring many shampoos before it is completely washed out. (See: "Henna" on page 39).
This is what you do to remove Henna from your hair faster.

Step 1: Start with clean dry hair. Put alcohol (70% proof) all over your hair and leave it on for 5 minutes. Soak up the alchol with cottonwool, making sure it doesn't drip and use it to apply the alcohol on the hair. Section the hair by making parts and applying it on each section.

Step 2: Fill an applicator bottle. Now put castor oil on your hair, over the alcohol (you can buy it in the drugstore). Sit under a hot dryer or use a heating cap (if you don't have either put on a shower cap) and wait for 15 minutes.

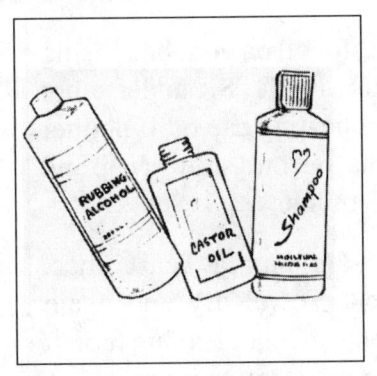

Step 3: Shampoo your hair at least once, rinsing well. Towel dry and apply rubbing alcohol again for another 5 minutes. Shampoo, rinse well and apply a creme rinse. This method is not damaging to your hair. Neither the alcohol nor the castor oil is capable of lifting the cuticle (outer layer of your hair) which would be damaging. Because this method removes the moisture and natural oil from your hair, you will need to apply a creme rinse afterwards.

Correcting Undesirable Hair Colors

How to Remove Metallic Dyes (Grecian Formula) From Your Hair

This type of hair coloring product is considered a progressive dye, meaning that every time it is applied it becomes darker and darker. (See: Metallic Hair Dyes on page 51). If after using this type of product you want to tint, bleach or perm your hair, you will first need to eliminate the metallic salts. Metallic salts are not compatible with the chemicals found in tints, bleaches or perms. Consequently your hair might turn pink or blue during bleaching, smoke or become very hot during hair coloring and turn copper/red if permed. Although metallic dyes are often difficult to remove from hair, you can try this method.

Step 1: Start with clean dry hair. Put rubbing alcohol (70% proof) all over your hair and leave it on for five minutes. Saturate cottonwool with alcohol and apply it on your hair. Section the hair and apply it systematically to each section.

Step 2: Now put castor oil on your hair, using an applicator bottle. Sit under a hot dryer, use a heating cap or, if neither are available, put on a shower cap and wait for 15 minutes.

Step 3: Shampoo your hair at least once, rinsing well. Towel dry and again apply rubbing alcohol leaving it on for five minutes. Shampoo, rinse and apply a creme rinse. This method is not damaging to your hair. Neither the alcohol nor the castor oil is capable of lifting the cuticle (the outer layer of the hair) which would be damaging. It will, however, remove the moisture and natural oils from the hair and therefore you will need to apply a creme rinse afterwards.

Correcting Undesirable Hair Colors

After you have completed this process you will need to make sure that all of the minerals have been removed from your hair.

Step 1: Buy a small bottle of 20 volume peroxide, clear household ammonia and an eye dropper (these items can be found in the drugstore). In a glass measuring cup, mix 1 ounce of 20 volume peroxide with 20 drops of clear household ammonia.

Step 2: Cut a strand of hair from the back of your head and dip it into this solution. If the hair gets hot, dissolves, develops a strange smell or quickly changes color from dark to light, it means that there are still metallic salts in your hair. If this is the case, you will have to repeat the removal process. Once all of the minerals have been removed, you can perm, tint or bleach your hair.

Answers to 10 Common Questions

Can Coloring Your Hair Damage Your Hair?

To begin with, the human hair is a very strong fiber, much stronger than most of us realize. Its physical and chemical composition make it possible for us to constantly wash, dry, perm and color it. The type of hair colors that dry your hair are tints (permanent color) and bleaches.

There are however different degrees of hair damage. Hair that is slightly damaged tangles when wet. Severely damaged hair tangles a lot, becomes matted and has a spongy feel to it. It loses all of its elasticity and will not hold a shape. This kind of hair is on the verge of breaking. Today it is rare to see such damaged hair. For hair to reach this stage of destruction requires tremendous abuse in the form of continuous over-bleaching (using a bleach that is too strong). You can tell to what extent hair is damaged by holding a strand on each end and gently stretching it. A healthy or slightly damaged hair will be harder to break than a very damaged one. A tint will slightly damage your hair but even this can be minimized by using the right application technique. (See: "How to Apply a Tint on page 43). Let me explain why permanent hair colors and hair bleaches can damage your hair. In order to understand this, you will need to know a little about the chemical composition of hair.

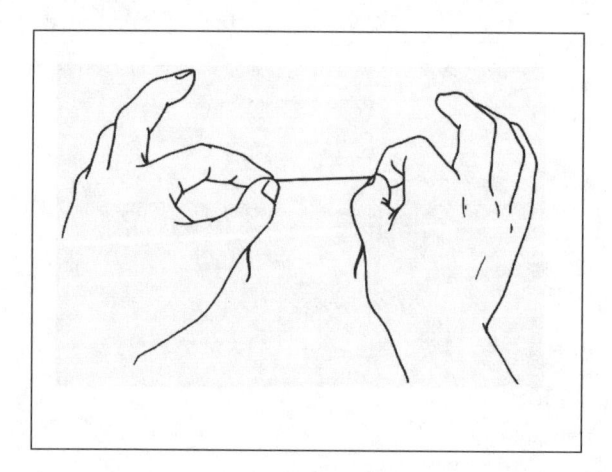

Answers to 10 Common Questions

The Chemistry Of Your Hair

Hair is 97% protein and grows an average of one-half inch per month. A hair may live two to six years before it falls out and is replaced by a new hair. We lose between 50 to 100 hairs a day with each hair being pushed out by a new one. The outer coating of the hair is called the cuticle which consists of a layer of overlapping, horny scales. The cuticle serves to protect the inside of the hair and is hydrophobic or water-resistant. These scales lie totally flat on the first two inches of the new growth, giving this part of the hair the most sheen. As the hair grows longer, and as the result of constant washing, drying, coloring, etc., the scales of the cuticle start protruding. A sure sign that this has happened is when hair is difficult to comb through after a shampoo. In this case, the hair is slightly damaged. The layer underneath the cuticle is called the cortex. It is hydrophyllic or water-absorbent. When the cuticle starts to peel away, it exposes the cortex. This kind of hair takes longer to dry because it absorbs more water. The cortex is the main segment of the hair and consists of protein chains which give hair its elasticity and bounce. Next you will need to know what exactly causes hair to become damaged. This depends on the degree of the pH value in the products you use on your hair.

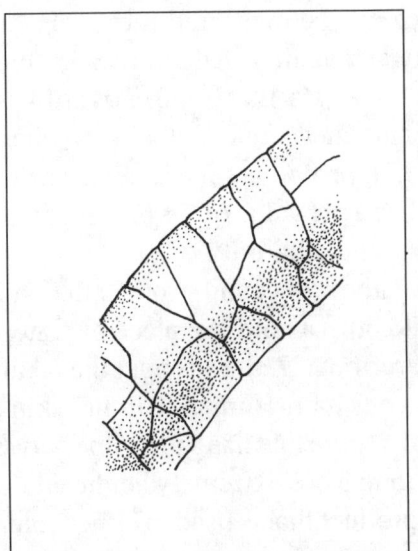

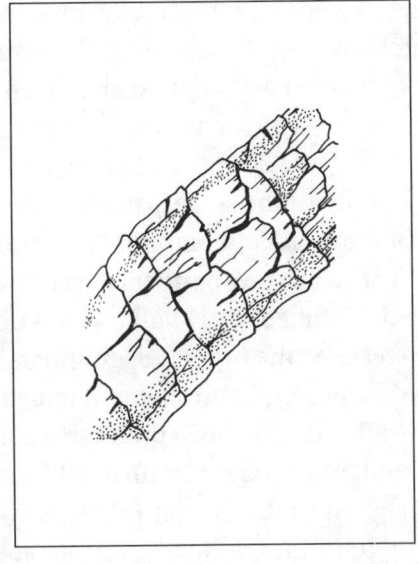

Answers to 10 Common Questions

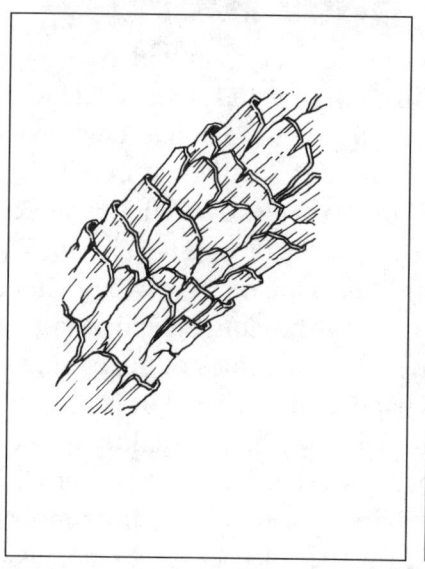

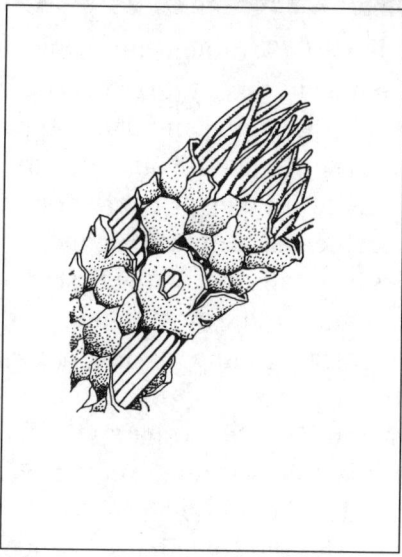

What does pH mean?

Every substance you use on your hair, be it a shampoo, hair color, peroxide, bleach, permanent wave or conditioner, has a different pH value. Every water-soluble substance can be measured for its pH value which means measuring its alkalinity and acidity. Alkalinity and acidity are measured on the pH scale. The pH scale starts at 0 and ends at 14. One side of the scale consists of approximate measures of alkalinity whereas the other side of the scale consists of approximate measures of acidity. The center of the scale is neutral and has a pH value of 7 which means that it contains an equal amount of acidity and alkalinity.

The lower the numbers are below 7, the higher and stronger the acidity is. For instance, a pH value of 1 would burn a hole in a piece of material. Conversely, the higher the numbers are above 7, the stronger the alkaline level is and the more it can damage your hair. Human hair and skin are naturally coated with a protective acid mantle that has a pH value between 4.5 and 5.6. Products with a pH less than 3 are extremely acidic and will damage the hair. Currently, the only product that is used to either color or perm hair that is acidic is an acid permanent wave. Different hair

Answers to 10 Common Questions

coloring products have different alkaline levels, depending on their different purposes. The stronger the alkalinity, the more damaging it is for your hair.

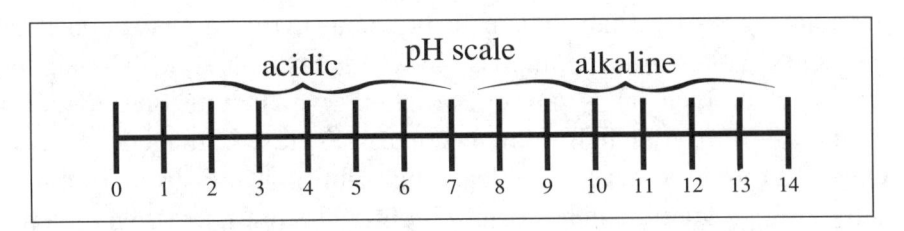

```
         acidic     pH scale    alkaline
    ├──┼──┼──┼──┼──┼──┼──┼──┼──┼──┼──┼──┼──┼──┤
    0  1  2  3  4  5  6  7  8  9  10 11 12 13 14
```

Shampoos have an approximate pH value of 7, permanents have a pH value between 7.5 and 8, permanent hair colors have a pH value of approximately 8, and semi-permanent hair colors have a pH value of about 7. Hair bleaches have the highest pH value, between 8.5 and 9. Both water and peroxide have a pH of 7. You can test the pH of products you use with Nitrazine papers which are available in the drug store. When you insert one of these papers into a shampoo, color, etc. it will change color indicating the pH value of the particular solution.

Answers to 10 Common Questions

Why do Permanent Hair Colors and Bleaches Need to be Alkaline?

The alkaline in a tint or a bleach opens the cuticle of the hair so that the coloring formula can change the pigments in the hair and deposit new pigments. This would be impossible without the alkaline. The alkaline level in a hair bleach has to be even higher, given that its job is to remove pigments from your hair. Hair becomes severely damaged when it is bleached too often, when the bleaching solution is too strong (too many activating powders which are very high in alkaline), or when the entire hair is bleached each time (except for very short hair). If you were to look at such hair under the microscope, you would see the cuticle standing up and in some cases non-existent, exposing the inside layer of the hair. The hair would feel spongy, lack elasticity and be very difficult to comb. After the remaining tint or bleach has been rinsed out, the cuticle will not lie flat but will continue to protrude. You will be able to tell because it will be difficult to comb. Hair after it has been shampooed is fly away but damaged hair is even more so.

Answers to 10 Common Questions

Can a Tint Make Your Hair Fall Out?

Definitely not! A tint cannot make your hair fall out nor is it even strong enough to make your hair break off. A tint is never the cause of hair loss. Internal reasons are responsible for hair that falls out. A tint solution cannot penetrate the scalp and thereby interfere with the growth of the hair.

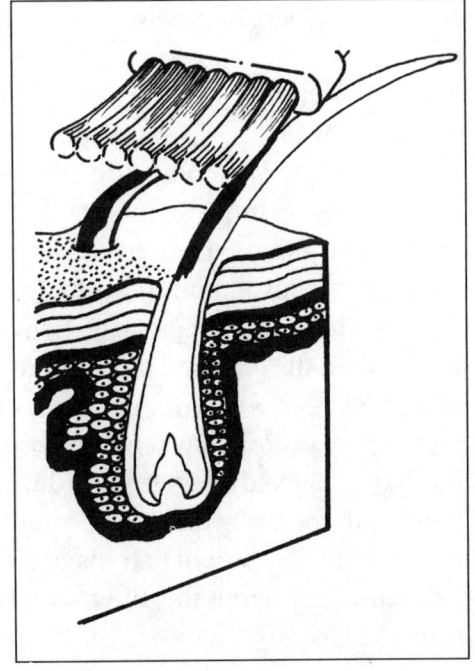

Answers to 10 Common Questions

Processing Time For Hair Color: How Important Is It?

Allowing your hair color to process for the required amount of time is very important. If the hair color is not left on your hair long enough, the coloring process will be interrupted and the color will be incomplete. Semi-permanent hair colors are usually left on hair for 20 to 30 minutes. Permanent hair colors usually need 30 minutes. Some permanent hair colors will start to look very dark after about 5 minutes, even if the shade is very light such as an extra light blonde. Although this may frighten you and you may want to immediately wash off the color, you shouldn't. The full processing time (30 minutes) is necessary to change your color to an extra light blonde. Hair colors are programmed to be on the hair for a specific amount of time after which time the coloring process is completed. So don't interrupt the process. Leaving a hair color on for a few minutes longer than the required time will do your hair no harm because once the color process has been completed it cannot have any further effect on your hair. Many years ago when tints were still new and unsophisticated, a tint had to be checked every minute during the processing time. Leaving it on your hair for even one extra minute could have meant the difference between having brown hair instead of blonde hair. Fortunately, we don't have to worry about this anymore. Hair coloring products have become safe and easy to use.

Answers to 10 Common Questions

How You Can Tell How Much White/Grey Hair You Have.

Follow the same procedure outlined in "How You Can Determine What Level Your Hair Color Is". If you look at the roots and notice the pigmented hair first, then you have anywhere from 5% to 50% white/grey hair. However if you notice the grey hair first, you will have anywhere from 50% to 100% white hair. Hair that is 80% to 100% white will look like a solid white color. When the white and the dark hair are equally mixed, the color will look grey.

Dark hair which has 30% to 50% white hair is described as salt and pepper. Hair that has less then 30% white hair still has pigmented hair as the most dominant hair color.

Perming Colored Hair

Hair that has been colored with a semi-permanent rinse can be permed with a perm solution intended for normal hair. Since the perm will remove some or all of the semi-permanent color from your hair, you should perm your hair first and then color it. You can perm your hair and use a semi-permanent color the same day. Hair that is colored with a permanent color (tint) should be permed with a perm solution for tinted hair. The same rule applies for streaked and highlighted hair. Because the process of perming (neutralizing to be precise) makes the color a little lighter, you should color your hair after the perm. Although it can be done the same day, waiting a day gives your hair a little rest. If the first 2-3 inches are straight (regrowth) and the rest of the hair still has perm in it, you should have a root perm. This will eliminate frizzy ends and not damage your hair.

Answers to 10 Common Questions

How Often Should You Tint Your Hair?

Permanent hair color (tint) can be applied as soon as the re-growth appears which is usually after about two weeks. Keeping in mind that a tint contains chemicals, it is best to wait as long as you can before coloring the re-growth. Of course this may not be possible when the contrast between the natural color and the tint is too visible. You can also minimize drying out your hair by applying the tint formula on the re-growth only each time you color your hair. In this way, you can avoid repeatedly coloring the same hair. (See: "How to Apply A Tint" on page 43).

How to Care for Colored Hair

The two substances most effective on damaged hair are a creme rinse and a protein conditioner. The chemical make-up of a creme rinse is such that its positive charges neutralize the negative charges in the hair and prevent hair from being fly away. When the creme rinse is applied, it attaches to the hair on contact. The positive charges in this substance combine with the negative charges of the hair. Technically speaking, this is known as an electrophyllic attraction. A creme rinse also lubricates the hair, making it easy to comb. A creme rinse should be applied after every shampoo.

A protein conditioner has a chemical make-up similar to that of a creme rinse but with one major difference - it contains hydrolized protein (Amino acids - proteins broken down to a certain molecular size in order to attach to the hair). An effective protein conditioner is one that has at least 18 amino acids present. Since hair is made up almost entirely of protein, the only substance that has any real re-constructive effect on its structure is hydrolized protein. The best strategy for keeping your hair in good condition after a tint or bleach is to apply a good protein conditioner once a week as well as a creme rinse after each shampoo. Although there is no visible difference after using a regular shampoo on tinted hair, manufacturers market shampoos specifically for colored hair.

Glossary

BASE COLOR
This term describes the color of your hair before applying hair color. Whatever color you start out with - be it your natural hair color or a color that was previously applied to your hair - is your base color.

COLOR LEVEL
The degree of lightness or darkness of a hair color indicated by numbers on a color chart.

TONE
The warmth or coolness in a hair color.

SHADE
Small degrees in basic hair color levels.

ASH
No red or gold visible in a hair color.

COOL
A hair color that has no visible red or gold tones.

WARM
A hair color that has red or gold tones.

RE-GROWTH OR ROOTS
The line that separates the new hair growth from tinted hair.

COMPLEMENTARY COLOR
Colors opposite each other on the color wheel. Complementary colors neutralize each other.

pH SCALE
A scale that indicates the acidity or alkalinity of a substance. 1 to 7 is acid; 7 is neutral; 7 to 14 is alkaline.

Glossary

CUTICLE
The outer layer of the hair. It is made up of transparent horny cells that overlap one another.

CORTEX
The middle layer of the hair underneath the cuticle. The medulla is the inner layer.

HAIR SHAFT
The portion of the hair that projects from the scalp.

ELASTICITY
The extent to which a hair can be stretched and returned to its original shape.

DAMAGED HAIR
A hair condition characterized by a dry lifeless appearance, tangling and a spongy feel when wet, lacking elasticity.

DEVELOPER
The substance that provides the oxygen needed to develop and oxidize permanent hair colors.

LIGHTENING ACTIVATOR
A substance added to the bleaching mixture (bleaching and developer) to increase the strength of the bleach.

TONERS
Provide the final color pigments on pre-bleached hair.